# Child Psychiatry Observed

Publisher's Notice to Educators

## THE PERGAMON TEXTBOOK
## INSPECTION COPY SERVICE

An inspection copy of any book published in the Pergamon International Library will gladly be sent without obligation for consideration for course adoption or recommendation.
Copies may be retained for a period of 60 days from receipt and returned if not suitable. When a particular title is adopted or recommended for adoption for class use and the recommendation results in a sale of 12 or more copies, the inspection copy may be retained with our compliments. If after examination the lecturer decides that the book is not suitable for adoption but would like to retain it for his personal library, then our Educators' Discount of 10% is allowed on the invoice price. The publishers will be pleased to receive suggestions for revised editions and new titles to be published in this important International Library.

# SOCIAL WORK DIVISION

*General Editor:* JEAN NURSTEN

Some Other Titles Of Interest

# Child Psychiatry Observed

a guide for social workers

Elizabeth Gore

PERGAMON PRESS

OXFORD · NEW YORK · TORONTO
SYDNEY · PARIS · BRAUNSCHWEIG

Pergamon Press Ltd., Headington Hill Hall, Oxford

Pergamon Press Inc., Maxwell House, Fairview Park, Elmsford, New York 10523

Pergamon of Canada Ltd., 207 Queen's Quay West, Toronto 1

Pergamon Press (Aust.) Pty. Ltd., 19a Boundary Street, Rushcutters Bay, N.S.W. 2011, Australia

Pergamon Press SARL, 24 rue des Écoles, 75240 Paris, Cedex 05, France

Pergamon Press GmbH, Burgplatz 1, Braunschweig 3300, West Germany

---

Copyright © 1976 Elizabeth Gore

First edition 1976

**Library of Congress Cataloging in Publication Data**

Gore, Elizabeth.
    Child psychiatry observed.

    (The Pergamon international library : social work division)
    Bibliography: p.
    1. Child psychiatry. I. Title. [DNLM: 1. Child psychiatry. WS350 G666c]
RJ499.G68 1975      618.9′28′9      75-6926
ISBN 0-08-017277-6
ISBN 0-08-017278-4 pbk.

---

Printed in Great Britain by A. Wheaton & Co., Exeter

*To*
*Mildred Creak*

# Contents

# Introduction

This book aims at an overview of child psychiatry written from the viewpoint of a clinical child psychiatrist. It is based on my experience in child guidance and child psychiatric clinics, but also on teaching contacts with social work students both in the clinical setting and in University seminars. Students have suggested to me, for example, that they find difficulty in linking the different aspects of their training in child development and child psychiatry, and that their reading often confuses them still further since exponents of particular schools of thought write tendentiously and disregard or denigrate other viewpoints. Often they cannot see the wood for the trees.

I have attempted therefore to make a linkage between different schools of thought in regard to normal and abnormal child development, clinical picture and treatment, dealing in some detail with those derived from psychoanalysis but also those based on learning theory. The experiences of certain children and their families are followed in the clinical setting during assessment and treatment, in order to bring life into the presentation and to point the practical application of what is being studied.

I have devoted a relatively large portion of the book to the subject of treatment. In fact the original idea came from a student who asked me to write a book called 'What is he doing in the playroom?' since he felt that few students have the opportunity of observing treatment in action or indeed children during assessment, and there was a need to remove some of the mystery. From this came the idea of taking the lid off child psychiatry and viewing it as far as possible as a whole and from the outside looking in.

Planning a book is rather like budgeting money. You have only so many words to spend, and if you spend lavishly on some aspects you have less to spend on others. Priorities are bound to be decided to some extent by the orientation of the writer. So although I have attempted to cover important schools of thought and research findings fairly, I have dealt in more detail with topics of which I have particular experience or interest and about which

I am presumably able to write with greater fluency. Sometimes a subject has been dealt with in detail because it makes important points which have wide application or includes work with other disciplines or is of particular topical and general concern. Failure to attend school (Chapter 8) fulfils all these criteria.

One question which concerned me was where should be the cut-off point in regard to age. Should this be a book solely about child psychiatry with the cut-off at the onset of puberty? This would tie in with the fact that adolescent psychiatry is on the way to becoming a speciality in its own right. On the other hand since the standpoint here is work in clinics to which school age children come (add to that preschool children and those staying on after the statutory school leaving age) this seemed arbitrary and from the clinical viewpoint unsound since many clinical entities, for example school refusal, spill over into adolescence.

I have decided to deal mainly with children up to the age of 12 but have also included something about early and middle adolescents where appropriate.

A further economy has been that I have not gone into details about how social worker students should apply the information in their own work. I am hopefully assuming that social workers with different orientations will read this book and that it will be more fruitful for them and for their tutors to apply the material to their own needs and experience.*

I still had to decide where to start. An easy way would have been to start with clinical entities, and this has some merit since it is certainly true that children who are troubled and children who are in trouble need help, and that to offer inappropriate or 'blunderbuss' help may result in 'do-gooding' without doing any good. Therefore, as in any medical speciality, assessment and diagnosis are essential; yet when the patient is a child, finding the meaning hidden behind what is overt may be of even greater importance for without meaning we have labelling without prognosis or without a guide to treatment.

So questions need to be asked about the origins of the symptoms or behaviour which the child shows, or which families show, the factors which perpetuated it in the past and those which are keeping it going. Thus we look

---

*I have adopted a numerical system of references. As some students may not have access to all the sources, alternatives have been added to the bibliography at the end of each chapter. Some of these are unnumbered and have been inserted in the appropriate place in the numbered bibliography. Other alternatives have been numbered in the text, providing an extra source.

Works marked with an asterisk are felt to be seminal material which students should try to obtain if possible.

at the child's early life, the family situation past and present, the school situation. It is necessary to distinguish between those factors which are immutable (mainly organic and constitutional), and those which can be changed or ameliorated (mainly developmental and environmental).

Happily the age-old controversy between nature and nurture is becoming less acute and many child psychiatrists and researchers prefer to emphasize the 'fit' between the child and his family and his environment (or the emphasis may switch entirely to the family). This more fruitful approach also takes into account that just as the bones of the child remain flexible and will bend rather than break so, except in rare instances of serious physical or emotional trauma, the feelings of the child are flexible and responsive and that maturation will usually contribute to the on-going development of childhood.

All this gives child and family psychiatry a hopeful and favourable orientation.

We start then by looking at child and family psychology and pathology. This will make the sections dealing with diagnosis more meaningful and help us to understand the problems of the children and families seen in our clinics.

### PART I

# Developmental Tasks and Hazards, Pathological Aspects

*The importance of the early years of life for healthy emotional development has long been established. It is claimed that the Jesuits considered the first 7 years to be paramount, and the poet Wordsworth expressed the same view when he wrote 'the child is father to the man'. Today such divergent groups as the psycho-analysts and the behaviourists lay stress on this period, although their emphasis differs.*

*Each stage in a child's development has its own tasks and hazards, needs and opportunities. Some periods are more stressful than others either because the stage of development itself is critical (some prefer the word 'sensitive') or because the parent is vulnerable in regard to that stage; for parents vary in the pains and pleasures they experience as they relive their own childhood through their growing child.*

*Each stage in development requires certain facilities and favourable experiences and if these are seriously lacking the loss cannot often be made up later. The needs of the infant are very different from those of the toddler or school entrant or adolescent, but the whole process is continuous and the successes and failures of each stage are cumulative and set an indelible seal on the personality of the child. Where failures or damage occur very early in life the effects are likely to be long-lasting, e.g. in severe emotional deprivation of the infant.*

*One modern contribution is the emphasis put upon influences starting even before what Susan Isaacs called 'the Nursery years', i.e. during prenatal life.([1]) Far from 'trailing clouds of glory', the infant carries the legacy of past maternal (and paternal) experiences, plus his own genetic endowment and acquired constitutional characteristics.*

Methodology

*By dealing fully with the first years of life, we are stressing the importance of this period for future development. It is necessary therefore to have a clear idea about the scientific status of statements about infancy.*

*Although precise statements about infantile experiences are often made, we must accept that they may be empirical. They have often been reached by reconstruction from present behaviour by the observation of the behaviour of psychotic and regressed children or by the retrospection of older children and adults undergoing psychoanalysis. Many such statements do, in fact, seem to fit the results of the more modern observational methods.*

*Observation of the pre-verbal infant, which has been developed particularly during the past 20 years, is probably the only reliable technique, though even here observer bias may reduce objectivity and the presence of the observer in the field must change the situation to some degree.*

*Infants have been studied in natural settings (among their families in their homes or foster homes) and artificial settings (clinics, hospitals and institutions) and some of these studies are utilised in this section, as are retrospective studies, and it behoves the reader to distinguish between them.*

*Where research findings are mentioned in this section, and throughout the book, the student is advised to study these in the original whenever possible. They will then realise that research methods and results must be scrutinised closely, since different research findings related to the same subject may be at variance with one another.*

---

CHAPTER 1

# Psychobiological

### A. Pregnancy and Birth

So we begin even before the nursery years with pregnancy, which is an emotional as well as a physiological preparation for motherhood. Changes in the mother's feelings have been well described by Helene Deutsch.([2]) Ideally, during pregnancy the woman's femininity becomes expanded to encompass the growing foetus with enough left over to include the father in shared experiences and positive phantasies. During this narcissistic state of wellbeing many women claim that they feel happier and more contented than ever before.

Not every woman is prepared practically or emotionally for motherhood. Physical illness, poverty, overcrowding or a large existing family may make the new pregnancy unwelcome, as may unplanned pregnancies especially when the parents are very young, immature or wishful of consolidating their future before starting a family. Unmarried mothers or women living at odds with their husbands may welcome the coming child for emotional reasons, but reject it because of social pressures. Relatively elderly parents conceiving after a long gap may feel totally unprepared. A 42-year old woman told me 'We had nothing for him; I don't mean cots or prams, you can borrow these, but feelings.'

Motherhood calls for maturity as well as femininity, it tests rivalries and defences and reveals submerged guilt. Many women, because of their own depriving experiences or because of the way in which the feminine role has been presented to them, feel inadequate both as wives and mothers. They may see the whole process from coitus to childbirth as suffering, pregnancy as shame, labour as terror and the puerperium as weakness and discomfort.

Not for them are the expansive phantasies of pregnancy, but instead frightening thoughts of a flawed child, or a baby as bad as they feel they were themselves. Such a mother may turn from her normal healthy baby and other adverse reactions may appear later. Childbirth is a highly subjective experience. The length of the labour, the difficulties encountered, the observed suffering of the women have little to do with the emotions the mother experiences both during the labour and after. Much depends on whether she regards the experience as rewarding or as unfair suffering. In this she is influenced by the picture given to her by her own mother, and by her general attitude to her bodily functions.*

## B. Stage of Symbiosis

During the first weeks of life, there is a continuation of the symbiotic state of the womb, and terms like 'the unity' or 'the nursing couple' have been used. J. Robertson ([3]) sees the mother's role as being 'a protective shield', and D. Winnicott who depicted the stage in such great detail called this 'the

*The effect of a number of variables, including prematurity drugs administered to mother during labour, anaesthetics, duration of labour, obstetric procedures, etc., on the first contacts between the neonate and his mother have been assessed by paediatricians, psychiatrists and others. It was found that contact by touch and eye contact, breast feeding and general bonding were all diminished by the situations and procedures listed.

holding phase' and viewed the mother's role as a 'caretaking' one. By this he meant far more than mere physical ministrations; it encompassed 'the whole environmental provision'. Winnicott[4] wrote of 'the good enough mother' who provides out of her own motherliness 'an easy and unresented pre-occupation with the one infant and an empathy with his need'. This 'good enough' person need not be the infant's own mother, and she may 'use a bottle for the feeding', but she must be able to accept all the infant's urges, first dependent but later aggressive; and she must supply all the oral satis-factions he seeks — not merely sucking, but also licking, blowing, smelling, touching and biting.

It is in this early state of omnipotence and egocentricity that the infant perceives the mother as part of himself and views her interests as his own. Winnicott[5] postulated that the infant feels that he has created the mother when he finds her there satisfying his needs.

Alice Balint,[6] writing of the same quality, says: 'the love for the mother is originally a love without a sense of reality, the child feels that the mother could not want anything which might run contrary to his wishes. It is an almost perfect counterpart of the mother's love for the child'.

Winnicott[7] felt, like Spock, that most mothers are 'good enough' if left to their own feelings and hunches, though his frequent use of the expression 'when all goes well' seems to suggest that there are times when things go less than well. He emphasised that success in maternal care depends on empathy and not on intellectual enlightenment.

The same conclusion was reached by Sylvia Brody,[8] who studied the nursing situation as it existed for each 'couple' in great detail and then attempted to gauge the mother's attitudes and feelings and the mutual satis-factions of mother and child during nursing. She found that a positive quality of satisfaction was only achieved where the mothers were truly sensitive to their infant's needs, and that their unconscious motivation for their choice of method and their latent attitudes to the total mothering situation affected the way the infants experienced the nurturing.

J. Robertson[3] studied well-baby (infant welfare) clinic records and followed the development of the infants. He found that the outcome was successful where the mother feels satisfaction not only in owning a child but also in the activities of mothering.

### Problems of fit between mother and child, 'Normal' discrepancies

Merril Middlemore[9] who from first-hand observations 'first saw the inter-twined richness of the nursing couple' noted what seemed to be inborn behavioural responses of babies, some being from the start lusty and active, others lethargic and passive. Mothers also varied in their response, some responding positively to the active lively infants, others to the passive contented ones. Feedback either positive or negative between mother and child was then observed.

S. Escalona,[10] who pioneered the study of 'well babies' in their families by studying them in their homes, pointed to the subjectivity of the infant's experiences, very different actions on the part of the mothers having a similar impact on the infants while similar actions had different consequences. Babies showed idiosyncrasies from the very beginning.

When all goes well her motherliness enables the woman to accept differences in response but vulnerable or immature mothers may be unable to do so. They may cherish an idealised picture of an infant who will be responsive and 'cuddly' and cannot see a contented undemanding child as lovable. Mrs A. who had adopted Sarah found her an 'unresponsive and quiet baby. She didn't need me', she added. But of her 'own' child Molly she said revealingly 'when I had finished feeding her or when I got up to her when she cried in the night, I felt that we were both satisfied.' Mrs B. on the other hand, an intelligent professional woman who needed reassurance that she could satisfy her child, might have coped well with the placid Sarah but she collided with a crying hyperactive baby who was difficult to comfort and love. Mrs B. retreated into an irritable depressive state.

Escalona in particular has stressed the importance of the fit between mother and child, and considers that this 'does away with the futile controversy as to whether infantile pathology is due to inadequate mothering or to inborn defect in the child'. Mothers, so apt to blame themselves, may take heart from this.

*Serious lack of fit, 'the basic fault'*

This was M. Balint's name for 'A considerable discrepancy between the infant's bio-physiological needs, and the material and psychological care available.'[11] Either the mother may be unable to provide 'the average expectable environment' or the infant may be unable to use it.

*Faults in the child*

The puerperal mother is particularly sensitive to anything unusual or unexpected in the infant's response. We have seen that the baby may be too exacting (for that mother) or too undemanding. He may show personality traits which she finds disturbing because of problems of her own. Even minor complications such as prematurity, a baby with a temporarily misshapen head, or one which does not suck, may rob her of her first tender response to the baby, and set going a train of anxious reactions, leading to a chain of negative feedback between mother and infant, and failure of bonding.

More serious complications such as severe subnormality, brain damage or physical illness of the child may prevent the development of rapport. Feeding is so central to the whole interaction between mother and child that if anything goes wrong with this it affects the whole relationship.

*Faults in the mother*

'Normal' reduction in provision not amounting to failure may be due to drain of emotional resources from the demands of husband or children, or to the mother's own emotional needs. Complications of pregnancy or childbirth may reduce the mother's ability to give warmth, and depression may do so in a more marked way. Personality disorders will have a more long-term effect.

The resulting care may be insufficient, inconsistent, haphazard, over-anxious, overstimulating or simply un-understanding, i.e. not responding to the infant's cues.

Escalona considers that a lack of basic experiences (bad as well as good) is the damaging thing, and results in a state of deprivation which prevents the infant from recognising his mother or mother substitute as a distinct person, and from forming a selective tie to her. D. Burlingham and A. Freud[12] have called this a 'deficiency disease', and many clinicians have pointed to later difficulties in forming relationships.

*Father's role*

We have seen that in most women there is a narcissistic regression to further the continuance of the pregnancy; in the man the biologic root is usually an instinctual drive for survival and the assertion of virility and manliness. During his wife's pregnancy his phantasies will be coloured by her attitude but also by his own experiences with his mother and father, and his ability to become a parent are closely related to these. He may envy his wife her creativity, feeling that his part was so quick and unnoticed. (It is quite different in some primitive tribes, where the husband helps to 'grow' the baby especially during the early months of pregnancy.)

Today, many husbands make use of the opportunity to be present during the labour, and to share with their wife the arrival of the baby. If the child is male this gratifies the father's instincts, and he identifies readily with his newborn son, but is also reminded of his own father. The amount of care of the baby which the father seeks and is allowed varies. Some mothers wish to do everything for their infants themselves, and some fathers feel scared of or alien to the fragile infant. Yet in many fathers the presence of the immature helpless baby produces a wish to nurture. This may be most important if there is a temporary situation where the mother, perhaps because of depression is unable to give adequate care and love.

There seems in any case to be more sharing of roles these days, as shown in the study of Newson and Newson,([13]) and the father also has a role to play during the symbiotic stage, by supporting 'the unity', by spending time with the siblings, and, as we have said, making up to the baby for any lack of maternal warmth.

Mr A. was able to empathise with Sarah's need for affection as an infant, and when Sarah became a toddler he found her an imaginative companion, while Mrs. A's awareness of the lack of rapport between herself and the child enabled her to seek help for them both. Alice Balint, however, emphasises the basic difference between the child's love for the mother and his love for the father, and claims that even when the father has assumed many maternal traits, 'the archaic bond linking mother and child is missing'. This has, however, the advantage that the child's relationship with father is more in accord with the reality principle.

These things have to be said in order not to paint too black a picture of chances of damage to the infant. Babies have two parents, and also grandparents, other family members and neighbours, all or any of whom may to a varying extent offset faults or failures in the mother, by becoming 'good enough' mother substitutes, or parents. It is where both parents in the absence of supportive or relieving 'others' are unable to provide the average expectable environment that danger looms.


## C. Separation-Individuation

*Weaning and distancing*

Winnicott([14]) stressed that the adaption of the mother to her baby's needs should be 'near perfect', and he saw her task as 'gradually to disillusion the infant so that he comes to recognise an environment which exists independently of himself'. He needs to see his environment as on the whole favourable and predictable, but there needs to be some frustration and change. Successful weaning, which means more than mere termination of breast or bottle feeding, depends mainly on the mother's ability gradually to distance herself from her infant which in turn depends on her sensitivity to the world outside her infant's needs.*

A. Freud([15]) has pointed out that it is difficult to draw a line between necessary frustration leading to individuation, and rejection, and she considers that even when the mother does not in fact reject the infant an excessively demanding baby may feel rejected, and may react in an extreme way as he senses a withdrawal of his mother's feelings from himself because of other claims on her emotions. When rejected, he feels inadequately loved; when mother withdraws, less loved. She considers that all kinds of behaviour on the part of the mother may be seen as rejecting by the child and regards disappointments and frustration as being inseparable from the mother-child relationship at every stage. Either mother or child may resist weaning. Where the mother has accepted ambivalence and individuation the infant is usually able to accept weaning and while mourning the lost object he finds pleasure in new ways of feeding and later in other childhood pleasures. His attitude to weaning can be seen as a blueprint of his attitude to changes of all kinds.

### Aids to individuation, transitional objects

Winnicott did not invent the transitional object, but he put his own personal stamp upon it. He wrote:([5])

> The transitional object represents the infant's transition from a state of being merged with the mother to a state of being in relation to her as something outside and separate. The gradual disillusionment . . . of weaning gives the infant an opportunity of developing an intermediate area of experience which originates out of illusion (that he has created the mother's breast out of his own need). From this area comes the transitional object, the infant's own thumb, a piece of cloth or old blanket, a ball of silk or a piece of string . . . of great value to the child as a defence against loneliness or anxiety especially at bedtime or when the circumstances of his life cause him to feel insecure and anxious, and parents are aware of this. It is important that the infant's rights over the object are respected that it is not altered in any way or taken away from him even if he is relatively old. It has to survive all kinds of treatment and feeling directed to it from the child. There may be a

*A. C. R. Skynner uses a striking analogy to delineate the concept of ambivalence; the child is like an object on the surface of the earth, bound to the mother by the force of gravity, hate is the fuel necessary to fire the rocket (child) into orbit by overcoming the gravitational force of love. Ambivalence is achieved when there is a confident balance between love and hate with movement towards and away from the object of attachment.

gradual shift away from the original object to a soft toy with a gradual extension of the range of interest, and the transitional object gradually loses its meaning, but may be sought again in troubled times.

Eventually the 'space' is left free to be filled by all kind of cultural and creative activities and by play.

## D. Progressive Individuation and Socialisation

As their child climbs through the successive stages of childhood both parents are presented with new adaptive tasks and the surviving threads of their own childhoods are in continual transaction with their growing children. As the child develops skills of locomotion, control over his bodily products, and speech, the mother in particular is confronted with each maturational event either reliving her own successes or regressing in the face of threat. The gradual emotional distancing of the child (and fathers are often better at accepting this than mothers), the development of relationships with siblings, extended family and the outside world, culminating in starting school, mean an increasing exposure of family patterns and problems. Parents may feel threatened by this and may deny quite ordinary difficulties. Or they may resent becoming part-time parents and identify strongly with the child, becoming unduly concerned about outside influences. Parents who cannot let the child go communicate their separation anxiety to the child and set the scene for problems such as school refusal, while others from their own resistance to authority (including school) cause maladaptation and rebellion.

Socialisation, by which is meant fitting in with the mores of the family and later of the outside world, develops from the favourable experiences of the child in his family. From his early experiences with his mother he learns to feel trust or mistrust, and from gaining some measure of bodily control, postponement of gratification and sharing. Spitz has stressed that from then on the presence of a predictable person (usually the mother) and the security she provides, 'her dos and don'ts and other communications both verbal and non-verbal open the door to all varieties of socialised activities' (the range depending on the mother's attitude).[16]

### Confused signals and double-bind

Clear communication between mother and child is clearly of great importance and Spitz and Lidz[17] both stressed the need for predictability in the communication and signals given to the child. Lidz has pointed out that words have a personal meaning for the child, from his own experience, as well as a family meaning, and that a marked discrepancy between the two may give rise to confusion leading to emotional incoherence; confusion over non-verbal meanings could have the same effect.

The best-known work has come from the Palo Alto group (Bateson *et al.*[18]) and has produced the concept of the 'double-bind'. This is a specific concept and should not be used loosely.

There are three requirements.

1. The involvement of two or more persons in repeated experiences concerning a primary negative injunction (usually verbal) with a second injunction (often non-verbal) conflicting with the first.
2. Both negative and positive injunctions are enforced by punishments or signals threatening survival.
3. The 'victim' is trapped by a final negative injunction prohibiting escape from the field.

It has been claimed that 'double-bind' behaviour is particularly important in the genesis of schizophrenia, but it may also be seen in the behaviour of mothers towards children who have developed other disturbances, e.g. school refusal. In Boston a recent study matched fifty schizophrenic patients who had attended the Judge Baker Clinic as children, with fifty non-schizophrenic patients who had attended at the same time. It was found that double-bind behaviour was more common in the mothers of the disturbed children who did not become schizophrenic in later life.

It seems that though double-bind is established as a pattern of behaviour, and has a pathogenic significance, this may not be specifically in the genesis as schizophrenia.

### E. Adaptation to Life Outside the Family. Middle Childhood

The period from somewhere between 5 and 7 and lasting until the onset of puberty at about 11 or 12 (known in psycho-analytic terminology as the 'latency period') has been considered to be a relatively 'quiet' time with the heat of the feelings centred round family life damped down and the child stretching out to embrace new experiences and relationships. Freud considered that the resolution of the Oedipus complex,* in his view the central struggle of childhood, freed instinctual energy to be attached (cathected) to new objects and situations, and that the relative suppression of sexual drives

*See Chapter 2, A.

helped to make this redistribution of libido (known as sublimitation) possible. Sublimation is considered to be important for social integration, intellectual curiosity and creative activities, and this period is thought to be the optimum time in the child's life for the development of new skills and knowledge.

Freudians would also consider that strengthening of the ego and the development of the superego ('the heir to the Oedipus complex'), as well as the beginning of identification with the parent of the same sex are important at this time. Phantasy and daydreaming give a release but may also act as a threat.

Where the conflicts of early childhood have not been resolved, or if sublimitation has not been achieved, defence mechanisms are likely to be formed and may assume a life style for the child, also behaviour problems appear.

This would accord with what one observes of children, who certainly at this stage seem to be very busy being little boys and little girls, finding roles for themselves individually and in groups outside the family, which is now needed mainly for background support, but also with the fact that problems are shown by referrals to child guidance clinics climb steadily during the second half of this period (other factors may account of this). It is also clear from studies by Rutter, Ford and Beach that sexual interests do persist.*

Problems may develop because of factors within the child, factors in the environment or interaction between the two.

We can see how the relative fragility of the child's self (ego) and the precariousness and incompleteness of his personality integration, plus residual conflicts from early childhood, render him vulnerable. His life outside himself offers opportunities for sublimation, but also a challenge which may be threatening. He has to cope with a number of quite complex and often stressful situations without the immediate support of his parents. If he has not already done so, he has to master the skills of caring for himself, to get on with a much larger number of boys and girls than he has met hitherto. Later he has to master 'the three Rs'. The success of his individuation, depends on the parents' attitude to this and to the advent of school, and also on the school itself, which allows or disallows gradual introduction of the child to this new environment, and especially the attitude of his first teacher. From his relationship with her and her relationship with him and with his family may stem his subsequent attitude to school and to learning.

Failure to conform to social requirements may be the first complaint from the school, and a child of 5 plus may be referred because the headteacher wishes to exclude him, but later both parents and teachers may worry about

*See Chapter 2, A.

failure to meet educational requirements. If the child is of low or borderline intelligence, especially if he comes from an intelligent middle-class family, expectations are likely to be high and the child may find himself under pressure, and later rejected as unsatisfactory. Or behaviour problems owing to internal conflicts or the discrepancy between standards and attitudes at home and school may develop. Boys tend to act out their problems more, and more boys are referred to clinics, but this may indicate a teacher bias as well as a tendency to refer children with disciplinary problems. Girls present more subtle disturbances.

## F. Adolescence

A brief reference to adolescent development and disturbance is included here to tie up with clinical studies, usually of early adolescents, appearing throughout the book.

Adolescence has sometimes been called 'the second spite period'; the first spite period being middle childhood when Oedipal and other conflicts are to the fore. In adolescence the thrusting physical and intellectual growth, and the surge of sexual feelings with emotional growth often lagging behind, make for a period of considerable storm and stress for both the adolescent and his parents.

Adolescence had been thought of as a clear-cut period, but an advance was made by D. Miller who subdivided it firmly into early adolescence (with links with early childhood), middle adolescence (search for identity) and late adolescence (search for role).[19] This fits well with the kinds of disturbances which the child psychiatrist may encounter at these stages.

The early adolescent may present unresolved childhood disorders which are little different from those of late childhood, or damped-down conflicts may emerge. Or strivings for independence in an over-protected and conforming child may arouse guilt, which may show as overt anxiety, school refusal or acting out behaviour. However this very striving for autonomy may cause improvement in neurotic disorders. Conduct disorders on the other hand tend to worsen, and children who have lacked parental attention and affection may become very unstable and rebellious.

In the middle stage problems 'typical' of adolescence may appear. These are usually connected with adolescent ambivalence, and with what has been described as an inner looseness and incoordination, leading to swings of mood and emotion and acting out.

In late adolescence problems more akin to adult disturbances, neurosis, depression and schizophrenia may appear.

The stages are not clear-cut and merge into one another. Indeed a characteristic of adolescent disturbances is that as well as being stormy there is a swing backwards and forwards to earlier and later stages of development.

## Adolescent Ambivalence

This is a total ambivalence, in which opposing tendencies are shown in many aspects of feeling and behaviour. Thus exhibitionism and brashness march along-side shyness and self-consciousness, feelings of excitement and omnipotence with embarrassment and inadequacy, a need for belonging and for conformity with the group mores with a 'lone wolf' attitude and originality, sudden dependence with a 'touch-me-not' attitude, sensitivity or 'one-way' sensitivity with crude insensitivity, tenderness with cruelty and so on.

## Peer Group

The peer group is often viewed with suspicion by parents, teachers and others, and indeed supported by it the adolescent may find himself able to do many things he would lack the confidence to do on his own; some of these things may involve disapproved sexual or antisocial activity. Yet if the adolescent kept with those his parents would choose for him he might remain fixed in the pattern of late childhood, and if a heterogeneous mix did not exist there would be a too-sharp division into 'goodies and baddies'. The national and international contact which exists between teenagers today, through pop stars, cosmetics, clothes and records gives a more general and less threatening support.

Yet parents find themselves in a difficult position. If their children behave badly, or get into trouble with their chosen friends, they consider that they are being 'led astray'; yet the choice of peer group friends is not made by chance, but because there is something in these particular persons which strikes a chord and meets a need. Particularly for an adolescent who feels inadequate or unwanted, his 'mates' and identification with them and with the gang may be the only source of satisfaction which he has, and an attempt to interfere may spark off serious rebellion or cause withdrawal or illness.

## Confidant

The adolescent may find a particular confidant among the peer group but he is more likely to choose an adult outside his family to fill this important role. Parents may feel hurt that their child confides in someone else, but this kind of learning can give tremendous support to the adolescent and may to some extent offset other influences. Warren has suggested that this is a ready-made role for the psychotherapist.

### Generation gap

It seems strange that the generation gap is given as one of the problems of the adolescent stage; for adequate separation of the generations has always been one of the criteria for healthy family living. Adolescents do not want their parents to be like them or even to understand them. If there is a problem it is a problem which parents have; perhaps seeing their adolescent offspring as objects of envy, especially at a time when they, the 'caretaking parents', are 'on the way down'. Very young parents may feel more in tune with teenagers, but should not want to step into their shoes nor act as siblings.

Parents who live vicariously through their adolescent sons or daughters or who relive their own adolescences may be over-permissive or over-restrictive.

In early adolescence in particular, structure, firmness and support are still needed from the parents, and some adolescent testing out behaviour is aimed at securing the reassurance of parental care and love.

### Sexual problems

Adolescent sexual problems are often thought of in terms of too early sexual precocity, promiscuousness, teenage pregnancies, i.e. the positive problems. The negative problems are those which most worry the adolescents themselves; on the physical side, under- or over-development, early or non-appearance of menstruation (and seminal emissions), persistence of homo-sexual interests, general feelings of sexual inadequacy, and lack of confidence in initiating relationships with the opposite sex, often covered by brash behaviour and sexual jokes.

This is well described by Salinger.[20]

### Stereotypes

Anthony[21] has suggested that parents (and society) get the adolescents they deserve, and he has described, among others, the following stereotypes of adolescents.

1. As both a dangerous and an endangered object. There is a fear of the power and strength of the adolescent but also a need to protect him from premature exposure to the dangerous adult world.

2. As a sexual object. The sexuality of the adolescent stimulates the. sexuality of the parent.
3. As a lost object to which the parents try to hang on, or they may help the process of separation.
4. As a maladjusted individual, with adolescence seen as a state of acute dis-equilibrium.

Immature and unstable parents enhance adolescent problems, but Anthony also stresses the 'good' reaction to adolescence, where the stereotype is minimal, and parents can enjoy their children's adolescence without living it with them.

Helene Deutsch[22] considers that the trend has been for the generation gap to disappear. The image of the mature generation becomes indistinct when adolescents discover that their parents are involved in their own unresolved adolescent problems. In addition there is a protest against 'the system' or 'the establishment', with denigration of accepted (adult) values, and adolescents project their own shortcomings on the outside world, overcompensate for inertia and passivity by assertion, rebellion or even brutality. At the same time Deutsch states that there is an increase of self-awareness, resulting often in a degree of self-devaluation, which may be compensated by an increase of narcissism (self love). When this happens the adolescent is able to use his energy for creative work (in a wide sense), and this may protect him from premature emotional entanglements.

Deutsch outlines the main areas of adolescent conflict as: a need to re-activate early defences and to find new ones, in face of the intensification of sexual impulses. Anxiety often centres round masturbation, which, she states, should be considered normal during adolescence, 'yet it often arouses guilt and fears of madness or physical damage, and tends to shatter self esteem.'

Laufer[23] goes further, and considers that masturbation not only confirms genital primacy, but also helps in ego organisation through the attendant phantasies, except when these are regressive or take on a homosexual content, when the adolescent may fear that he is not normal. Then he may regard his body as his enemy, or alien to him, or feel that it is or could become out of his control. This may be very frightening. Blos sees the loosening of infantile ties which occur in adolescence as a 'second individuation process', and many writers see this period as the last opportunity to find a solution to the Oedipal conflict.

Anna Freud[24] stresses the normality of the devaluation of the parental image, and many other aspects of adolescent behaviour; for example it is normal for the adolescent 'to rebel against his parents, and to be dependent on them, to love them and to hate them, to be more idealistic than he will ever be again, but also to be the opposite, self-centred, egoistic, calculating'. She advises that adolescents be given time and scope to work out their own solutions, while realising that parents need help to accept the difficulties they will have in their attempts to liberate themselves. The rebellion against parents will be all the more spectacular if there has been a strong parental fixation, and in these cases the first choice of a love object is likely to be a homosexual one.

Adolescent conflicts cannot be seen in isolation, but in relation to infantile experiences, and success or failure in dealing with environmental hurdles. This point is stressed by Erikson,[25] who sees the task of the adolescent as a search for identity in the following ways; finding a working role, the acquisition of social attitudes and opinions, separation from the parents ideologically and in fact, and definition of the sexual role. Success leads to the development of a sense of identity, failure to 'role diffusion'.

### Bibliography and Further Reading

Items marked * are particularly important sources. Unnumbered references provide alternative sources to the reference quoted immediately above.

*1.    Issacs, Susan (1929) *The Nursery Years,* Routledge & Kegan Paul, London.
       Isaacs, Susan (1933) *Social Development in Young Children: A Study of Beginnings,* Routledge & Kegan Paul, London.
 2.    Deutsch, H. (1946) *The Psychology of Woman,* Research Books, London.
 3.    Robertson, J. (1962) Mothering as an influence on early development, *Psychoanal. Study Child* 17, 245–264.
 4.    Winnicott, D. W. (1965) *The Maturational Processes and the Facilitating Environment,* Hogarth Press, London
 5.    Winnicott, D. W. (1951) Transitional objects and transitional phenomena, in *Collected Papers.* Tavistock Publications, London.
 6.    Balint, A. (1939) Love for the mother and mother love, in *Primary Love and Psychoanalytic Technique* (ed. Balint, M.) (1952) Hogarth Press, London.
*7.    Winnicott, D. W. (1957) *The Child and the Family,* Tavistock Publications, London.
 8.    Brody, S. (1956) *Patterns of Mothering,* International Universities Press, New York.
*9.    Middlemore, M. (1941) *The Nursing Couple,* Hamish Hamilton Medical Books, London.
10.    Escalona, S. K. (1963) Patterns of Infantile experience and the development process, *Psychoanal. Study Child* 18, 197–244

11. Balint, M. (1968) *The Basic Fault*, Tavistock Publications, London.
    Spock, B. (1956) *Baby and Child Care*, Pocket Books Inc., New York.
12. Burlingham, D. and Freud, A. (1944) *Infants without Families*, International Universities Press, New York.
*13. Newson, J. and Newson, E. (1963) *Infant Care in an Urban Community*, Allen & Unwin, London and Penguin Books.
    Newson, J. and Newson, E. (1968) *Four Years Old in an Urban Community*, Allen & Unwin, London.
14. Winnicott, D. W. (1956) Primary maternal preoccupation, in *Collected Papers* (1958). Tavistock Publications, London.
    Bowlby, J. *Maternal Care and Mental Health*, W.H.O., Geneva.
*15. Freud, A. (1965) *Normality and Pathology in Childhood*, Hogarth Press, London.
16. Spitz, R. A. (1957) *No and Yes*, International Universities Press, New York.
    Warren, W. (1952) In-patient treatment of adolescents with psychological illnesses, *Lancet* i, 147–150.
17. Lidz, T. (1964) *The Family and Human Adaptation*, Hogarth Press, London.
*18. Bateson, G. et al. (1963) A note on the double bind: 1952, *Family Process* 2, 1, 154–161.
    Bateson, G. (1960) Minimal requirements for a theory of schizophrenia, *Archs. gen. Psychiat.* 2, 477–491.
19. Miller, D. (1969) *The Age Between*, Cornmarket, Hutchinson, London.
    Warren, W. (1965) The psychiatry of adolescents, in *Modern Perspectives in Child Psychiatry* (ed. Howells, J.), Oliver & Boyd, Edinburgh.
20. Salinger, J. (1951) *The Catcher in the Rye*, Penguin Books, Harmondsworth.
21. Anthony, E. J. (1970) The reaction of parents to adolescents and their behaviour, in *Parenthood* (ed. Anthony, E. J. and Benedek, K.), Little, Brown & Co., Boston, pp. 307–324.
*22. Deutsch H. (1968) *Selected Problems of Adolescence*, Hogarth Press, London.
23. Laufer, M. (1968) The body image, the function of masturbation, and adolescence, *Psychoanal. Study Child* 23, 114–137.
24. Freud, A. (1958) Adolescence, *Psychoanal. Study Child* 13, 255–278.
25. Erikson, E. H. (1959) *Identity and the Life Cycle*, Psychological Issues, International Universities Press, New York.

## CHAPTER 2

# Theories of Child Development

I have represented the views of the different schools as objectively as possible, and have purposely used technical terms where these have specific meanings. Application of some of the material will be found throughout the book. Where this is appropriate I have attempted to make links and applications, and in regard to the behaviourist school, have included some details about treatment.

## A. Psycho-analytic

### 1. Infantile sexuality

This is one of Freud's important but often misunderstood contributions. Certainly it exploded the 'myth' of childhood innocence, but was intended to mean much more than mere genitality, including every activity of early childhood aimed at obtaining local pleasure (the feelings aroused called 'libido') from a particular organ or area 'erotogenic zones'. The child is said to be 'polymorph perverse' in that pleasurable feelings are aroused by activities which in adults would be seen as abnormal, (such as fetishism, cruelty, exhibitionism.)

In the oral stage, the infant gains pleasure from all kinds of mouth activities (sucking, bubbling, licking, mouthing, biting). In the anal stage pleasurable sensations are aroused from urination and defaecation, and from playing with urine and faeces, offset by demands made for the control of these functions. When the child's experiences with the mother are on the whole favourable he is thought to internalise a 'good relieving mother'. He certainly needs a good relationship with this all-important and all-powerful person to help him to accept, for example, that she only values his bodily products at certain times and in certain places, and that she expects him as time goes on to share her and his possessions and to delay gratification.

T. Main([1]) has described most vividly what happens when a 'bad' mother is internalised. The infant's phantasies are of 'biting teeth, scratching fingers, piercing genitals', to be countered by his own 'burning urine, exploding faeces, poisonous flatus'.

Starting at about 3 years of age (the genital stage), as part of a growing curiosity about people and the world about him, the child may show a particular interest in sexual differences and roles, while his intense feelings about his parents and siblings lead him to spontaneous enquiry and activity.

Gradually more direct feelings and desires take the place of purely auto-erotic sensual pleasures, and while masturbation increases, marked hetero-sexual preferences are shown ('Oedipal' and 'Electral' situations). The mother may be embarrassed by the little boy's overtures to her (he may fondle her breasts and want to get into bed with her) and the father irritated by the boy's hostility to him, but where marital relations are strained or the father often away the mother may secretly be gratified by her son's preference.

Much depends on how parents cope with this stage. When parents feel a need to suppress masturbation and sexual curiosity the boy may become anxious and if specific threats have been uttered, he may fear an attack on his penis especially if he is aware that girls do not possess one ('castration anxiety and complex'). This could lead to inhibition of feelings and curiosity in a wide variety of activities with a pleasurable content, and even a loss of assertiveness and aggressiveness. If the mother can avoid being seductive and the father punitive, yet stand up as a male to his son's aggressiveness while tolerating his sexual strivings, rivalries may be smoothly resolved, and by the age of 7 and the beginning of latency, the father can offer himself as a model to his son for identification.

The girl too will have phantasies about the anatomical differences she has noticed, which may lead her to believe that her penis was taken from her as a punishment, or that her mother failed her in not ensuring that she had one. This would be an additional reason for her to turn from the mother to father, and to look to him for the satisfaction she believes her mother to have. It is important that the girl can see her mother as an appreciated and feminine person gaining satisfactions from her role as a woman, or she may fail to identify with her, instead remaining jealous of the male ('penis envy').

*Sexual enlightenment of children*

Three aspects of the child's own experience involve him in speculation about sexual functions; the pleasure he has found in the manipulation of his own genitals, his observations of male and female differences, and the observed behaviour of his parents. He (or she) feels very muddled, but it is not sufficient for a parent to give factual or diagrammatic representations (rather than stories about storks or gooseberry bushes). It is essential to take into account the level of part-knowledge and phantasy which the child has reached. Both boys and girls during the stage of preoccupation with anatomical differences tend to assume that the presence or absence of a phallus alone makes the difference. When interest switches to curiosity about the origin of babies girls may have phantasies of oral impregnation (by kissing) and both sexes may believe that babies can be made by urination or by exposure of the male genitals. Later phantasies centre round the method of expulsion of the foetus (now known to be carried in the mother's body) which is often thought to take place through the naval or anus.

Parental reticence and embarrassment about sexual matters, plus the child's own observations, sometimes including the primal scene, may lead him to see sex and coitus as shameful or sadistic. Because of this and because of his own 'love affair' with his parent he may be unable affectively to accept the information given, unless he can see that his parents are capable of accepting the pleasures that sexuality can provide. This does not mean excessive display or stimulation but calmly accepting sexuality as truly one of the facts of life.

### Events in relation to stage of libidinal development

It is the way a child experiences an event which determines the effect it has upon him. Psycho-analysts claim that if for example the father is hospitalised when the boy is at the height of the Oedipal complex he may develop anxiety (shown by fears or phobias) while a male sibling born at this time would be seen as another rival for the mother's love.

### Recent research

Some confirmation for this material originally formulated theoretically or gathered from analyses can be found in recent research. There is also a change in emphasis.

Rutter,[2] from his study of spontaneous conversations of young children and their answers to questions, found corroboration of the general Freudian view of infantile sexuality, though the stages were blurred, with oral activities continuing during the whole of the preschool period. In another study he found that attitudes towards childhood sexuality were passed from one generation to the next, and that sexual identity was closely related to the sex assigned to the child. Ford and Beach[3] found that in permissive societies sexual interests persisted right through 'latency' with masturbation, homosexual and heterosexual play showing a gradual increase from 5 years onwards.

## 2. Anatomy of personality

Another Freudian concept was of a reservoir of unorganised basic drives (libidinal and aggressive) existing in the unconscious part of the personality. The drives (the 'id') which follow the pleasure principle seek expression in consciousness and in action. When the drives come up against the reality principles a conflict of purpose results and the 'ego' acts as a regulator exercising some control over the drives and bringing into play defence mechanisms to fend off anxiety. The ego also mediates between the subject and the outside world.

Gratification of primitive drives is also limited by the 'superego', which is formed in childhood by the internalised standards of the parents and which assists the process of socialisation.

The 'ego-ideal' is a more conscious development of the child's aspirations.

## 3. Defence mechanisms

Although defence mechanisms are used by children, they are less skilled in their usage than are adults and therefore more at the mercy of anxiety engendered by drives which are unacceptable to ego or superego.

*Denial.* The child refuses to face the facts of reality and even the evidence of his own misbehaviour, replacing them by phantasies or wish-fulfilment.

*Repression.* The child refuses to allow unacceptable thoughts to reach consciousness, especially hostile thoughts, for example, about a baby brother; jealousy is denied or overcompensatory affection is demonstrated.

*Projection.* Here the hostile thoughts are projected and this has the advantage of allowing the child to see his own hatred and hostile behaviour as a result of the hatred of the other. Or the child may project his fear of leaving mother onto some neutral situation at school.

*Reaction Formation.* A strong but threatening impulse is converted into its opposite. Thus rituals, compulsions, and obsessive cleanliness replace destructive and sexual drives.

*Regression.* The child may turn from a stage of development where he is meeting obstacles to an earlier phase when he received gratification (commonly seen after the birth of a sibling).

Children tend to use one or two defence mechanisms exclusively. Much of the behaviour of children which causes bewilderment to parents and teachers is explained on the basis of defence mechanisms.

### 4. Coping mechanisms

These are considered by Anna Freud to be ways in which the child learns to deal with stress. They are much closer to consciousness and to reality than defence mechanisms, and also closer to normality. They create a kind of life style, but one which may modify or even change as the child grows older. Anna Freud looks upon them as healthy developments which have greater flexibility than the defence mechanisms which may become rigidly fixed, and she considers that they help rather than hinder the development of ego strengths.

### 5. Object relations and ambivalence

These are a part of distancing and individuation, of accepting first the mother, then the father, then 'important others' as capable of satisfying and frustrating, loving and hating, and of the child's ability to accept his own feelings of love and hate. This and his willingness gradually to postpone gratification is the beginning of the child's relationship with objects in the world outside.

### 6. Paranoid-Schizoid and Depressive Position (Melanie Klein)

These important concepts are closely connected to ambivalence and object relations. Klein[4] postulates that because of frustrating as well as satisfying experiences, the infant splits these with the 'good' objects being introjected and the 'bad' objects projected. The good and the bad cannot be held together at the one time, nor in the one person. This is an unintegrated stage which she has called (perhaps misleadingly) the 'paranoid-schizoid position'.

If experiences are mainly favourable this is progressively replaced by a more integrated state, 'the depressive position', when he recognises whole objects (the first one is mother) and accepts ambivalence in his feelings and hers. At the same time there is a greater awareness of his dependence on her and of himself as a person. The 'depressive' aspect arises because of the ambivalence and guilt which the infant feels in regard to his destructive impulses, and since he has begun to distinguish between phantasy and reality he cannot escape. Klein claims that the depressive position is never wholly worked through, and when there has been marked failure depressive anxiety is likely to be overwhelming at later stages. Or worse there may be a fixation at the earlier paranoid-schizoid stage. Rene Spitz[5] has described the depressive position in different words, as '8-month anxiety'. The relevance of the psychoanalytic viewpoint to treatment is detailed in later pages.

## B. Theories of Piaget [6,7,8]

These are the lifetime studies of a psychologist working in the clinical field, and comprise studies from birth to maturity of the developments of intellectual functioning.

Piaget has worked in two ways, by conducting free-ranging interviews with children, and by observing children's attempts to solve tasks set with concrete materials. His main interest has been in the way children think and develop concepts, through increasingly complex schemata of thinking from developing understanding of the physical world. Limits are set by the degree of maturation, and therefore one kind of thinking and behaviour is characteristic of each stage. Particular behaviour arises because of the way the world appears to the child, and it becomes organised into more general and complex patterns.

*Stages*

*Sensori-Motor* (0-18 months). The infant reacts to objects which are perceptually present and if he cannot see them he appears not to believe in their existence. He appears to assume that the objective world is centred round his activities, and that any change or movement in it results from some activity of his. As he learns to distinguish between himself and objects, he is able to see himself as one among other objects in his field and to relate to perceptually absent objects in that field. Piaget regards play at this stage as 'pre-symbolic' or 'practise play'.

*Symbolic and Pre-Conceptual* (18 months – 4 years). Objects begin to be represented by memory images, and he begins to form symbolic representations of the objective world, but everything centres on himself and his view of the world is more in accord with his needs than with objective facts. From a need to conserve his own identity he assimilates new events with past experiences, and affective reactions with previous feelings, but without accommodating them to reality. Thus he has a false view of reality. Make-believe play is part of this stage.

*Intuitive stage* (4—7 years). Accommodation to reality increases, with continual verification of statements by testing in action, plus correction of false beliefs. But changes in the state of objects confuse him, and he cannot take into account viewpoints in the physical world which differ from his own. His thinking continues to be egocentric and animistic, but there is gradual decentralisation of the focus of interest.

*Concrete-operational* (6—11 years). Thinking has become much more complex and sophisticated. There is increased objectivity and he can take into account spatial viewpoints other than his own, and deal with two variables at once. Accommodation (to reality) and assimilation (to his personal needs) are nearer equilibrium.

*Abstract-operational* (from 11 years). He can form abstract concepts and reason from hypotheses, so-called logical thinking.

*Relevance to Child Psychiatry*

Piaget's work has value as an objective clinical study of the development of intelligence in children, and forms a bridge between the intellectual, and the motivational-emotional aspects of development which are usually studied separately.

It complements but also acts as a corrective to the assertions of some of the other schools. Piaget's findings help to explain reactions in terms of the stage the child has reached, and may point to ways of handling and helping.

For example, with regard to hospital admissions; a very young baby who has not as yet formed memory images shows preoccupation with his physical environment on return home, while a baby of about 7 months he will show a disturbed relationship with his mother. The marked reactions of 2- to 4-year-olds are explained by the strong tie to the mother plus an inability to understand promises, and the view of the 6- to 8-year-olds that their illness is a punishment for bad behaviour accords with Piaget's findings on the moral judgments of children of this age group. (Psychoanalytic explanations for these would of course be very different.)

An important aspect is the egocentric and animistic view which the child has up to the age of 7. His belief that his thoughts and wishes can affect the movement of the sun, the moon and the stars, that the clouds follow him or that his shadow is part of himself give him feelings of power but may also be frightening. His belief that objects in his world have feelings just as he does builds a world full of menace especially as his own feelings are so strong. Leila Berg([9]) has described this in *Little Pete*.

Bobby was a shy boy who disliked school when he started at 4½. His mother, in an attempt to form a bridge between home and school, suggested that he should take some flowers from his garden with him. 'They would be unhappy there, like me. They'd shrivel up and die', said Bobby.

The less intense emotional reactions observed after 7 years may rest on better reality testing, with important figures seen as more real and less threatening.

Piaget's concept of a balance between assimilation (serving inner needs) and accommodation (serving reality) would explain the young child's tenuous grasp of reality, and suggest that emotional factors could cause delay in the development of accommodation. Any imbalance could cause maladjustment in social situations; excessive assimilation meaning a flight from reality with immature patterns of behaviour, and excessive accommodation and too-ready adaptation to reality with flawing of personal development.

Divergence from the psycho-analytic view is most marked on the question of memory, play and dreams. The dream is regarded by Piaget as pure assimilation in which contact with reality is lost.

## C. Theories of Erikson ([10,11])

Basic to Erikson's views is the concept that each stage of development and the success or failure in dealing with it sets a permanent stamp upon the developing personality, and that arrest at a particular stage ('fixation') may occur or the individual may return to an earlier stage in the face of stress ('regression').

He stressed the general links between childhood, adolescence and adulthood. Each stage of libidinal development carries also certain tasks of an emotional and social nature; in the oral stage they centre on trust and mistrust, and if there is a fixation at this stage, the positively fixated crave dependence through their lives, while the negatively fixated struggle constantly against dependency. In the anal stage the child has to achieve an acceptable arrangement with the powerful person(s) in his life; success brings autonomy, failure either excessive compliance or obstinacy, with a lasting feeling of doubt and shame. In the genital or 'initiative stage' the child has to reach a co-operative solution and some measure of autonomy without too much guilt. Success brings initiative, failure anxious withdrawal.

During latency permanent attitudes to work and to peers (colleagues and friends) are laid down, based on the individual's confidence in his capacity to 'do'. Here Erikson writes of industry in those who are successful and inferiority in those who are not. In adolescence the tasks include a search for identity and role.

Immaturity, whether due to fixation or regression is seen as a failure to solve the crucial interpersonal problem at one or another of the stage of development.

*Relation to Child Psychiatry*

Erikson postulates that failure to cope with stress evokes a need to regress to the point of failure, there to encounter the developmental challenge. Strength may be gained from the temporary return to a period of relative satisfaction and treatment should assist the attempt at surmounting the developmental hurdle. Failure to achieve this results in fixation.

Erikson considers that stress and mounting anxiety may be seen in a positive way as providing motivation to learn new skills and to utilise new methods of coping, and also that failure of defence mechanisms especially where these have been rigid and inflexible, can be utilised for re-education and the building up of more adequate defences. Families may do this for themselves, as shown by Anthony's([12]) study (p. 61) or may be helped by techniques such as crisis intervention (p. 217).

Erikson's theories have been useful in the treatment as well as in the understanding of adolescents, and have been the basis, along with the work of Piaget, in the formulation of a treatment scheme for delinquents (p. 84).

## D. Behaviourist School ([13,14,15]) (Psychological-physiological theories)

According to Learning Theory, child development is seen as proceeding through a process of conditioning, whereby desirable behaviour is reinforced by approval and undesirable reduced or extinguished by punishment disapproval or loss of love. By a process of generalisation and the labelling of classes of behaviour as 'good', 'naughty', 'clever', 'stupid', the child builds up a conditioned autonomic reaction to such classes of behaviour. Thus all behaviour is learned, adaptive as well as maladaptive.

The autonomic nervous system is important in that the sympathetic (fight and flight) mechanism or the parasympathetic (relaxation and contentment) are called into play in situations with a physical and emotional content. Childhood fears are explained by behaviourists on the basis of an initial fear reaction for example to a large barking dog or a strange noise, and become reinforced as the child avoids the dreaded confrontation. The fear may then spread to other similar situations concerning animals or even to a general fear of being out in the street. On the other hand, familiarity and facing up to the situation especially if the mother is able to remain calm and not feed into the child's anxiety may lead to extinction of the fear. This explains why many children 'get over' their fears (spontaneous remission). It is interesting that stress is laid on the effect of confinement (inability to escape from the field) in enhancing the fear reactions.

For the behaviourists there is no such thing as psychic conflict or psycho-dynamic causes of neurosis, Eysenck writes 'While the term symptom is used there is no evidence that it is symptomatic of anything. There is no under-lying complex or other "dynamic" cause; all we have to deal with in neurosis is maladaptive conditioning and behaviour.' At the same time behaviourists deny the criticism that they are only interested in getting rid of the symptom, since they are concerned about reduction of anxiety.

Eysenck distinguishes two types of maladaptation, one due to faulty conditioning and leading to 'personality' problems (fears, phobias, asthma), which is mediated by the sympathetic; and one due to lack of conditioning in which habits or behaviour which give pleasure to the individual are unaccept-able to society or are damaging to the individual (sexual deviation, fetishes, alcoholism, smoking) which are mediated by the parasympathetic.

There is a tie up here with Eysenck's concept of personality, in that the first group with neurotic-type symptoms appear in introverted persons, while the second group with conduct-type disorders in the extroverted. The first group show a tendency to remit spontaneously, condition well and respond to most forms of treatment; the second group are more resistant.

*Application to Treatment in Child Psychiatry*

*'Conditioning'.* This is included here for convenience, but in the examples given for the treatment of phobia, many child psychiatrists would consider psychotherapy aimed at uncovering underlying conflicts the treatment of choice. See also Chapter 8. This may be used in conduct disorders in children, usually with the aid of introverting drugs such as amphetamines, which render the child more responsive to conditioning. This may be by 'socialising con-ditioning' (under favourable situations this may be carried out in the home or

at school) or by 'operant conditioning', where positive or negative feedback (by rewarding or punishing) is given to the child according to the behaviour he shows.

In 'aversive conditioning' a severe type of punishment is used in such conditions as alcoholism, sexual abnormalities, and (originating from the United States but increasingly used here) in autistic and retarded children who show problems of behaviour and communication.

Treatment of enuresis by conditioning is dealt with in the appropriate section.

*'Deconditioning'*. This is used particularly in specific phobias and attempts to follow the pattern of a normal remission. A situation is set up whereby the child feels contented and relaxed, perhaps being seated on a comfortable knee and fed sweets. A 'hierarchy' which relates to the specific problem is planned, and presented to the child. For example, if the phobia is of cats, the child is first shown a picture of a kitten, then of a cat, then a toy kitten and a toy cat and finally a real kitten and a real cat. Systematic distraction or play situations may be added. A similar procedure may be used in older children with fears, where a hierarchy is presented starting with what the child considers to be the least disturbing aspect of the situation (with the child relaxed or under hypnosis) building up as the child becomes able to accept this to more and more stressful aspects. Eysenck has pointed out that this method is often used in school refusal where the school is presented to the child 'in small doses' and indeed he claims that behaviour therapy techniques are used in a variety of situations in child psychiatry without this being acknowledged.

*'Flooding'*. Here the aim is extinction of a response, when the noxious stimulus is repeatedly presented, and this is the rationale of treatment by flooding in phobias, sometimes called massed practice in tics. The most potent stimulus is presented; the result is alarm followed by adaptation as the stimulus is repeatedly presented. Relapses are claimed to be less common with this form of approach.

*'Intermittent reinforcement'*. This produces greater resistance to extinction than does continuous reinforcement. A child who cries at night when put to bed has the behaviour reinforced every time the parents go to her room or bring her downstairs. If the parents cease doing so for several days or even weeks the demanding behaviour becomes even more intense. As family members find it difficult to continue the withdrawal of attention which is essential for success, the presence of a social worker or health visitor in the home to give support to the parents and also to 'model' for them the part of a non-anxious adult in the situation may be required.

*'Modelling'.* This concept needs to be explained. Psychoanalysis stresses the importance of the unconscious modelling of parental, sex and gender appropriate behaviour (by identification, etc.). The reward this receives may be seen as reinforcement of the desired behaviour. Learning theory has further examined the modelling (or copying) which takes place outside the family, and which is particularly important for socialisation and peer-group modelling (for good or ill). Certain criteria for successful modelling have been worked out. The model should have a certain prestige or cachet, but should not be so far above or so different from the subject as to create a feeling of unease or alienation. The model should be seen to be coping and adequate rather than superior, and the behaviour which is to be modelled should be seen to be rewarded. The model is at his most effective when he is seen to be human, to have some failings and to exhibit feelings towards the subject, for example, warmth or hostility, and to show approval or disapproval.

Modelling can be useful in work with adolescents, and also with families when a frank 'no nonsense' approach helps the adolescent or the family to respond frankly and openly.

Thus in the example given above, if the social worker or health visitor appears too immaculate, perfect or efficient the parent will become too uneasy or anxious to carry out her role.

## Bibliography and Further Reading

Items marked * are particularly important sources. Unnumbered references provide alternative sources to the reference quoted immediately above.

1. Main, T. (1963) A fragment on mothering, in *Psychosocial Nursing* (ed. Barnes, E.), Social Science Paperbacks, in association with Tavistock Press, London.
*2. Rutter, M. (1971) Normal psychosexual development, *J. Child Psychol. Psychiat.* **11**, 4, 259–283.
3. Ford, C. S. and Beach, F. A. (1951) *Patterns of Sexual Behaviour*, Harper & Row, New York.
*4. Klein, M. (1957) *Envy and Gratitude*, Tavistock Publications, London.
5. Spitz, R. A. (1946) Anaclitic depression, *Psychoanal. Study Child* **2**, 313–342
6. Piaget, J. (1953) *The Origins of Intelligence in the Child*, Routledge & Kegan Paul, London.
7. Piaget, J. (1954) *The Construction of Reality in the Child*, Routledge & Kegan Paul, London.
8. Piaget, J. (1951) *Play, Dreams and Imitation in Childhood*, Routledge & Kegan Paul, London.
*9. Berg, L. (1959) *Little Pete Stories*, Puffin Books, Harmondsworth.
*10. Erikson, E. H. (1963) *Childhood and Society*, Norton, New York.

*11.  Erikson, E. H. (1959) *Identity and the Life Cycle,* Psychological Issues, Monograph 1 International Universities Press, New York.

12.  Anthony, E. J. (1970) *The reaction of parents to adolescents and their behaviour,* in *Parenthood* (ed. Anthony, E. J. and Benedek, J.), Little, Brown & Co., Boston, pp. 307–323.

13.  Eysenck, H. J. (ed.) (1960) *Behaviour Therapy and the Neuroses,* Pergamon Press, Oxford.

14.  Eysenck, H. J. (1962) Conditioning and personality, *Br. J. Psychol.* 53, 3, 299–305.

15.  Rachman, S. (1962) Learning theory and child psychology: therapeutic possibilities, *J. Child Psychol. Psychiat.* 3, 3/4, 149–163.

## CHAPTER 3

# Aspects of Deprivation

### A. Maternal Deprivation: Separation and Rejection

It is important to be clear at the outset that separation from mother need not be equated with deprivation, but that rejection if severe should be.

The first studies of young children separated from their mother were carried out by R. Spitz[1] and J. Bowlby[2] on children in institutions where there was adequate physical and hygienic care, but totally inadequate emotional care and parenting. Under these circumstances Spitz found for example that not only the newborn (thought to be most vulnerable) but also infants who for the first 6 months of their lives had experienced satisfactory relationships with their mothers and who were then placed in institutions showed a deterioration which was physical, social and emotional. They lost weight, their developmental quotients (D.Q.) fell, and they became susceptible to intercurrent infection. After a distressed weepy stage they became irritable and then withdrawn, showing finally a total lack of interest, rigidity and depression. Beginning socialisation seemed to be most damaged, with loss of previously acquired language and speech. Spitz found that when the condition had persisted for more than 6 months it was irreversible in the absence of special therapeutic measures, such as intensive mothering-type psychotherapy.

Bowlby linked similar findings with such long-term effects as development of an 'affectionless' character and delinquency.

Thus workers in the field were alerted to the dangers of irreversible damage being done as a result of long-term separation from the mother, and it is unfortunate that this was taken up so enthusiastically that any separation of mother and young child came to be thought of as harmful. Bowlby himself did not say this[3,4,5,6], and indeed his own later studies on children separated from their mothers under a variety of conditions indicated that it was the alternative provision which was all-important. He distinguished, for

31

example, between separation where 2-, 3- and 4-year-olds were placed full-time in an institution day nursery when the D.Q. fell and children of the same ages cared for in day nurseries while the mother worked, when D.Q. was normal.

Where, however, the alternative care was unstable or unsatisfactory the children began to show signs of disturbance. The same proved to be true of institutional care. Family grouping with a spread of ages was preferable to groups of the same age, especially where under 5's were concerned; and many people consider residential nurseries to be depriving, especially where job allocation, rather than child allocation, is the rule.*

James and Joyce Robertson([9]), as part of their study of young children in brief separation, observed and filmed a 17-month old child (John) from a secure home during 9 days spent in a residential nursery while the mother was in hospital to have a second child; and in a contrast study took into their own home a child of the same age (Jane) who stayed for 10 days for the same reason. They conclude and illustrate on film† that, contrary to much that is said in contemporary literature, the reaction of young children of 1½ to 2½ years to separation from the mother *per se* is anxiety but not necessarily acute distress and despair. The response depends mainly upon the quality of substitute care during the separation.

The fathers of John and Jane visited each day, but in other respects the circumstances were totally dissimilar. John was in an institution where the 'job assignment' system fragmented the care of the children, did not allow meaningful relationships to develop, and denied to John the understanding and protective mothering-type care that he needed. Since no nurse was assigned to him his needs were not recognised; he was not protected from the aggressive behaviour of the deprived long-stay toddlers who were his companions; foods and routines were strange; no attempt was made by the nursery to adapt to the rhythms and needs of this individual child.

For the first 2 days John tries to find a nurse to take the place of his absent mother, showing good expectation based upon previous good experience. But he is disappointed, turns in despair to seek comfort from teddybears, then slides rapidly downhill into acute distress and apathy. At reunion he cannot

---

*The whole controversy is well documented by Rutter([7]) and Wallston([8]).

†Robertson, J. and J. (1968). Film: *JANE, aged 17 months, in fostercare for 10 days* 16mm, sound, 37 min. Guide booklet. Concord Films Council, Nacton, Ipswich, New York University Film Library. (Also in Danish, French, German, Swedish.)

Robertson, J. and J. (1969). Film: *JOHN, aged 17 months, for 9 days in a residential nursery*. 16mm, sound, 45 min. Guide booklet. Available as above.

accept his mother, and turns away from her with hostility which is chilling to see. Over the next few years continuing repercussions of a negative kind are reported.

Jane, on the other hand, had been familiarised beforehand with the Robertson home and family and came into the care of a responsive substitute mother who had fore-knowledge of the child's habits, likes and dislikes, preferred foods, etc., and was fully available to recognise and respond to Jane's needs. It is not possible to talk to a child so young about the absent mother. But Jane was cared for in a way which maintained her experience of warm mothering, so that on reunion she went to her mother after only a moment's hesitation — smiling and with good expectations.

John was looked after in a setting in which the stress of losing the mother was grossly aggravated by additional adverse factors which cumulatively overwhelmed and traumatised — i.e. damaged — him. Jane was cared for by a responsive substitute mother in a benign setting. All her resources were therefore available to deal with the one stress that could not be eliminated — namely loss of the mother; Jane, therefore, did not deteriorate as John did, but was held in a state of 'manageable anxiety'. But the Robertsons are careful to point out that even with the best of care separation from the mother remains a hazard for young children because of the discontinuity on the interaction between mother and child. Despite the good care given to Jane there were subtle changes in her subsequent attitude to her mother[9].

It is clear from the Robertsons' writings and films that individual differences in response to brief separation from the mother are determined by the interaction of a number of variables. These are set out in Chart 1[9] which is reproduced by the kind permission of the authors.

## B. Hospitalisation

This is a special kind of separation in which the child finds himself not only in surroundings which are unfamiliar, but which may have a disturbing connotation for him because of previous experiences (Robertson[9]). He may be in pain, he may feel extremely ill. The procedures themselves may be painful or frightening. Operations on the eyes or genitals, severe burns and fatal or chronic illnesses are liable to be particularly upsetting to the child and his parents (who may need as much help as he does to deal with their guilt over an accident or a serious burn). Admissions at certain ages, or after the recent birth of a sibling may be upsetting.

Chart 1. *Factors which combine to determine individual differences in young children's responses to separation from the mother.* *

|  **A.** | **B.** |
|---|---|
| *Factors in addition to loss of the mother which are likely to cause stress.* | *Factors likely to reduce stress.* |

**A.**
*Factors in addition to loss of the mother which are likely to cause stress.*
1. Strange environment.
2. Inadequate substitute caretaker.
3. Strange caretaker.
4. Multiple caretakers.
5. Cues/language not understood and responded to.
6. Unfamiliar food and routines.
7. Unusual demands and disciplines.
8. Illness, pain, bodily interference.

9. Bodily restriction.

**B.**
*Factors likely to reduce stress.*
1. Familiar substitute caretaker
2. Known foods and routines.
3. Toilet demands unaltered.
4. Own belongings.
5. Unrestricted body movement.

6. Familiar environment.
7. Reassurance of eventual reunion.
8. Keeping apart fantasy and fact ('My Mummy doesn't love me').
9. Reminding child of parental disciplines.
10. Support from father.
11. Willingness of caretakers to talk about parents and previous life.

**C.**
*Child's psychological status which may increase or reduce overt distress during separation, may increase or decrease the overt upset after separation, may increase or decrease the long-term effects.*
1. Ego maturity, level of.
2. Object constant, level of.
3. Quality of mother-child relationship, facets of.
4. Defence organisation.
5. Fantasies about illness, pain, physical interference, disappearance of mother, etc.
6. Preseparation experience of illness/separation.

Arrangements for 'humanising' children's wards have been implemented in most hospitals. Daily and often unrestricted visiting, allowing the parents of young children to help with procedures and feeding, to be present at bedtimes, all help, as do increased stimulation, the provision of playthings (and play therapists), and allowing children home for weekends. However, it is not so much what is done, but how it is done; mothers need to feel welcome and useful on the wards. Some are rendered incompetent beside the efficient nurses who may tactlessly say, 'Here let me do it' to a struggling mother. By tradition the mother does not feel at home in the hospital setting, but this passes if she is given support.

The late Sir James Spence[10] would pose a question to each new Houseman as a baby was wheeled from the operating theatre into the sideward and placed in his cot, while the waiting mother sat on a chair in the corner.

*Reprinted from J. and J. Robertson (1971), Young children in brief separation: A fresh look, *Psychoanal. Study Child* 26, 264–315.

'Where should that baby be?' The wanted answer was 'In the mother's arms'. Some think that it is most important for the mother to be present as the child is going under an anaesthetic and as he comes round, but not all anaesthetists and not all ward sisters would wish this. It is often said that the child is more likely to be upset if the mother is there. This argument was often used against visiting: children 'settled' better if left without visits. They may have shown less upset but it seems likely that the 'settling' was in fact despair and apathy.

Studies have shown that children are helped by being encouraged to show their feelings of grief and fear, and that children between 2 and 4 who apparently settled well showed more disturbance later than those who showed distress, and that counselling of ward staff about this and the need for special comforting during procedures, lessened emotional disturbance during hospitalisation and even more markedly on discharge and follow-up.

Group staff assignment to individual children also lessened disturbance; in all circumstances, but particularly where the mother is unable to visit or to visit frequently, the young child needs to know to whom he can turn for help or comfort. This may be brushed aside by 'most of our mothers do visit', or 'They get too attached to the one nurse. They demand too much'. We must remember that the child whose mother does not visit is in a worse position than if visiting had never been introduced. (See also Prugh *et al.*[11] and Rie *et al.*[12]).

## C. Family Hospitalism

The child although living in his own family can become deprived. We can see how this could happen if the mother rejects him, but it may also occur if the serious pathology of one or both of the parents causes the child to be scapegoated by the whole family; his emotional development is delayed or deformed and he grows up with a feeling of frustration and emotional hunger. He seeks unlimited affection or shows apparent indifference and an inability to accept love.

Keith, aged 8, was the second child of a family of four. Both his parents had been brought up in institutions, and were immature, the father weak and passive, and the mother domineering but inadequate. She was able to accept her first child, a girl born when the parents were still receiving some support from their own families, but she disliked Keith from the moment of his birth.

They had recently moved from their home town, and Keith was born after a trying pregnancy and labour into a state of poverty and overcrowding. Mother recalled, 'Another male to look after'. I thought, 'He'll be just like his father. I wished I could put him right back where he'd be safe'. Keith was a very attention-seeking child, who was meeting rejection at home, at school and in his neighbourhood. A student remarked 'Keith seems to be the most disliked child I've ever met'. In the clinic he presented one ailment after another. On the first interview he gave me a list of accidents to himself, falls from walls and trees, knocked down by a car and a bus, nearly drowned, and finally 'A arrow in me eye'. One day he spied my lunchtime apple, ate it quickly and on the next visit complained because there was no apple and said he'd go and see the 'Doctor downstairs'. (Mother changed her family doctor at about this time.)


### D. Parents who Cannot Keep a Safe Home

*Non-accidental injury to children*

It was not by chance that Keith's mother made the remark that she wished she could put him back 'Where he'd be safe' (from her aggressive feelings). We are now considering parents who abuse their children physically or who allow repeated accidents to happen to them. This concept seems to be preferable than the very emotive term 'battered' to describe the babies or children, while the parents are 'battering'. For here again we see the cycle of deprivation in action. Such parents are usually young, immature and dependent and have little confidence in being lovable. They were often physically abused themselves as children, made to feel inept and worthless by their mothers. Now they tend to see adults as unhelpful people and their babies as bad (often an extension of their childhood selves).

In spite of this they usually start off with the hope of being good parents, and indeed the practical aspects of motherhood are often well carried out, the children being exceptionally clean and well clothed; but there is a lack of true motherliness. The contrast between the nutrition and clothing of the child and the attitude of the parent plus the string of accidents or injuries is marked. Or periods of good protective care may give way to times when phantasies get the upper hand and overwhelm the parent. In this situation there is a remarkable absence of guilt since the parent feels the action was inevitable. Usually only one parent is involved, but the other may be collusive.

In some instances the child himself may unwittingly stimulate the attack, for example a handicapped or coloured child. Jane was an unmarried girl who had had four illegitimate children by different men. She was intelligent and independent and all her children were beautifully dressed, but one (the first and the only coloured child) had sustained several fractures which Jane admitted she had caused. Jane came from a middle-class family; when she became pregnant her father was able to accept this until Jane told him the baby might be coloured. 'That would be the death of me' said the father, and on the day the baby was born he died of a heart attack.*

## E. Deprivation Syndrome†

This has been called by some 'a variant of battering'.

These babies and young children fail to thrive; their relatively large heads and pot bellies contrast with their small stature and matchstick limbs. Their extremities are blue and cold. They appear sad and depressed and lack energy.

These mothers too have been deprived; they seem unable to respond to this particular child, or there may have been a failure of bonding, or the mother may have a problem which affects the feeding, e.g. a fear of vomiting, or because of circumstances at the time of the birth.

The children improve in hospital, gain in stature, weight and animation but relapse on return home.

Under experimental conditions the children improve if given a basic diet plus extra stimulation, or if given a high calorie diet. If the mother is recommended to follow a particular diet at home (or the diet she says the child is receiving) there is no improvement, but if a worker goes to the home and gives the feeds the child improves. It appears that either the child does not get the diet the mother thinks (or says) he does, or he is unable to utilise it. A point of interest is that some of the mothers commented to the worker who gave the child his food, 'I did not know he could eat like that', which may suggest that 'modelling' on learning theory lines might help some of these mothers.

*Since the above was written two study groups have reported their deliberations on the question of non-accidental injury to children. In May 1973 The Tunbridge Wells Study Group[13] (Multidisciplinary) discussed Prevention, Recognition and Management, Team Work and Case Conference (including the vexed question of police involvement), the size of the problem, reflections on the parents, education and research.

†In December 1973 the findings of the Working Party of the Department of Child Health University of Newcastle-upon-Tyne were reported in the *British Medical Journal*[14] (three paediatricians, one child psychiatrist, the Director of Social Services and the Medical Officer of Health). They dealt, in general, with diagnosis, immediate action and further management, and a separate section detailed the management by the Social Service Department.

See also Helfer & Kempe,[15] Smith *et al.*[16] and Skinner [17].

As early as 1959 D. MacCarthy and E. Booth[18] began a study of ten children showing stunting of growth and reported their findings in 1970.

In the last three categories, we have situations which are potentially dangerous to the life and health of the child. It may be that at a certain point someone has to take the responsibility of saying, 'This child must be taken from his natural home for his own protection', but all concerned need to be able to say 'This parent needs help', without discriminating against parents whose behaviour is openly inimical to the child.

There has been a swing away from the more punitive attitude at least in the professional and helping agencies, although nurses may find it difficult to repress an emotive response to the parents of severely damaged children who come into their care, especially if there are several children from one family. The move is towards a more therapeutic but also a more scientific attitude. Studies within the group of parents rather than between these and other parents who do not damage their children or allow them to become damaged, look to be the most fruitful approach. Wide-ranging assessments of the parents including psychological tests seem likely to separate out a group of parents who have been so seriously deprived or damaged or in some other way faulted that they cannot respond to the needs of their child(ren) even after help on an intensive or long-term basis. In these cases the risk is too great if the child remains, and in some instances if the one child victim is removed another child is likely to take his place, so that all the children may have to be protected.

It is good news that the NSPCC has set up an advisory centre in London which will replace The National Advisory Centre on the Battered Child. This is first an emergency and follow-up treatment department, and centres are being set up in other cities. Research will be continued, and it is hoped that answers will emerge which will be a guide to selection of families for therapy.

### F. The Cycle of Deprivation. Disadvantaged Children

What we have learned about the causes and effects of maternal deprivation may help us in a study of a more total deprivation. Some children may be thought of as being handicapped from birth onwards by multiple disadvantages which interact unfavourably with one another and with the social set-up to produce a state of deprivation which tends to reproduce itself in generation after generation. In this context deprivation is seen as a lack of the essentials necessary for healthy physical and emotional growth; of needs rather than wants.

Aspects of deprivation may appear at all levels of society but 'the most vulnerable are those already at the bottom of the social ladder' (Sir Keith Joseph[19]). This fact was demonstrated convincingly by a study published in 1972 by the National Children's Bureau under the title *From birth to 7* (Davie *et al.*[20]). This interdisciplinary study of all children born in England, Scotland and Wales during one week of 1958 (the 1958 Cohort) demonstrated that by the age of 7 'serious and important inequalities have been established'.

Children whose parents held unskilled manual jobs were found at 7 to be more likely to

Have been born abnormally early or late, to be abnormally light or short.

Have squints, stammers or difficulty in co-ordinating their movements.

Be bedwetters or nail biters, to have suppurating ears.

Come from broken homes, and to have less well educated parents.

Despite the provision of remedies for the above, they are also:

Less likely to have been immunised or vaccinated.

Less likely to attend clinics or visit the dentist.

Less likely to have had physiotherapy.

More likely to have parents who are reluctant to consult teachers.

More likely to have homes which are overcrowded and lack normal amenities.

And the children are more likely to

Be aggressive and destructive.

Be maladjusted.

Reject adult standards.

Speak unintelligibly or have poor oral ability.

Have poor general knowledge, and be non-creative.

Do less well at school and be poor at reading and arithmetic.

Taking the first group, the first three points are connected with pregnancy and childbirth, and a study by the 'Bureau' on illegitimacy (Crellin *et al.*[21]) showed that at birth such children were usually first babies, of low birthweight, born to young mothers who had little or no antenatal care or attention at birth, (see Chapter 10). That such children, disadvantaged at birth, can catch up is shown by studies of those who were adopted, but most illegitimately-born children have to face an interacting network of adverse circumstances while they are growing.

The second group indicates how low-income group parents are less able to use important facilities, and the third group shows the results in lack of attainment (at 7 there is a gap between the most advantaged and the most disadvantaged of 4 years in reading attainment), and maladjustment. With the latter there is a strong link with delinquency as was shown by D. West ([22]) of the Cambridge Institute of Criminology. It is clear that this kind of deprivation operates in a cycle, but a cycle which is composed of a network of interacting forces.

It is not enough to point to overcrowded homes and schools and to poverty. For the findings of D. West cast doubt on the role of the purely physical environment in producing deprivation and multiple handicap. He suggests that families gravitate to the bottom of the class structure because they are inadequate and comments on 'the remarkable concentration of parental pathology, in the shape of unsuitable discipline, unfortunate attitudes to children, personality deviation among the disadvantaged group'.

The 1958 Cohort study showed children being unequally prepared for the race of life, and other studies suggest that they are not even being prepared for the same race (See Sears *et al.*([23]) and Newson and Newson([24,25])). For parents of each social class tend to prepare their children to be members of the class into which they are born, and each generation transmits a tradition of attitudes and behaviour to the next. Greater social mobility does not seem to have altered the attitudes of working-class and middle-class parents very much. Working-class mothers believe that the most significant actions arise outside her home, and see the world beyond her home and neighbourhood as alien and potentially catastrophic. She feels unable to influence events or the behaviour of her children which she sees as beyond her understanding. She looks more to the consequences of her child's actions than to the meaning beneath them. She wishes her children to grow moral and upright, but since she does not see parents as being able to achieve this, she looks elsewhere for authoritative help and guidance. Working-class fathers tend to opt out in the spheres of decisions and discipline, except at times of crisis, when both parents rely on physical punishment in the hope of maintaining law and order.

When we look at the attitudes of middle-class parents it is easy to see how for example schools feel more at home with these parents and find their children more rewarding. (This could be true of staff in Clinics too?)

For the middle-class mother sees her child's behaviour as complex and requiring understanding; she is more interested in intent than in action, and both she and father tend to be supportive and active. Both wish to expose their children to worthwhile experiences both at home and outside, and allow them to be self-directing. They look to a democratic solution to disciplinary problems and prefer symbolic to physical punishment. These parents are less likely to look for direct advice but are responsive to suggestions from experts in the fields of child care and education.

It must be axiomatic that education should compensate for disadvantage, and the Plowden Report([26]) proposed that resources should be concentrated on Educational Priority Areas, particularly deprived areas, considering that 'education is a social distributor of life's chances'. However this may not be enough for the researchers of the Halsey Committee([27]) and other studies have considered that although educational expansion had raised the level of attainments of the different social groups, it had not changed their relative position, and that 'the impact of the educational system on the life of children remained heavily determined by their family and class origins'. The Halsey research team found that 'most parents are profoundly interested in their children's education and social chances' but that the 'EPA' parents particularly are conscious of their inability to help their sons and daughters, and were themselves school failures both socially and academically. They do not see themselves as having a role to play in the education of their children, and the researchers concluded that 'social distances have to be traversed' because 'not only must parents understand schools, but schools must also understand the families and environment in which the children live', and moreover that 'schools should try to come to terms with the values of the community instead of implicitly opposing them'.

The need for this has already been shown by another piece of research which demonstrated that communication between home and school decreases progressively down the social scale (Douglas ([28])), as does the school performance of the children, so that by secondary school age the gap between the attainments of the disadvantaged children and the rest has widened markedly even among high-ability children, (see also Ryan([29])).

The recommendation of the Halsey researchers was for community-orientated education for the EPAs starting with nursery centres with links with the infant schools, but also using parental co-operation and local community involvement.*

---

*The experience of two members of the Woodberry Down Child Guidance Team, Mrs M. Boxall, Educational Psychologist and Mrs G. Gorrell-Barnes,([30],[31]) who worked in schools with nurture groups for deprived children and with groups of the parents respectively is relevant here. The children were of primary school age, and a high proportion were from immigrant families. They were referred to the nurture groups by the teachers on account of serious behaviour disturbances, and teachers from the school were invited to take the groups. It is postulated that the groups have a value in preventing future disturbance, delinquency and violence.

These findings and recommendations bring us back to the personal aspects of the cycle of deprivation; to the special needs of emotionally deprived parents who need help on their own account if they are able to meet the needs of their children. This help may have to be on quite a long-term basis, and while they are receiving this help they need to be living in a society in which 'parents and homes are supported, and not supplanted and overruled' (Halsey). Then these parents will see themselves as having a value, as having something to contribute, and as able to have some say in important matters in the lives of their children.

## Bibliography and Further Reading

Items marked * are particularly important sources. Unnumbered references provide alternative sources to the reference quoted immediately above.

1. Spitz, R. A. (1945) Hospitalism, *Psychoanal. Study Child* 1, 53–74.
2. Bowlby, J. (1952) *Maternal Care and Mental Health*, W.H.O., Geneva.
3. Bowlby, J. (1969) and (1973) *Attachment and Loss*, Vols. 1 and 2, Hogarth Press, London. Vol. 1: *Attachment* (1969); Vol. 2: *Separation: Anxiety and Anger* (1973); Vol. 3: *Loss* (in preparation).
4. Bowlby, J. and Ainsworth, M. (1956) The effects of mother-child separation: a follow-up study, *Br. J. med. Psychol.* 29, 211.
5. Bowlby, J. and Ainsworth, M. (1968) Effects on behaviour of the disruption of an affectional bond, in *Genetic and Environmental Influences on Behaviour* (ed. Howells, J.), Oliver & Boyd, Edinburgh.
6. Bowlby, J. and Murray Parkes, C. (1970) Separation and loss within the family, in *The Child in his Family* (ed. Anthony, E. J. and Koupernik, C.), Wiley-Interscience, New York.
   Yudkin, S. and Holme, A. (1963) *Working Mothers and their Children*, Michael Joseph, London.
   Mead, M. (1954) Some Theoretical considerations on the problem of mother-child separation, *Am. J. Orthopsychiat.* 24, 471–483.
*7. Rutter, M. (1972) *Maternal Deprivation Reassessed*, Penguin Books, Harmondsworth.
8. Wallston, B. (1973) The effects of maternal employment on children, *J. Child Psychol. Psychiat.* 14, 81–95.
*9. Robertson, J. (1958) *Young Children in Hospital*, Tavistock Publications, London.
   Robertson, J. (1962) Mothering as an influence on early development, *Psychoanal. Study Child*, 17, 245–264.
10. Spence, J. *et al.* (1954) *A Thousand Families in Newcastle-upon-Tyne*, Oxford University Press, London.
11. Prugh, D. G. *et al.* (1953) A study of the emotional reactions of children and families to hospitalisation and illness, *Am. J. Orthopsychiat.* 23, 70–106.
12. Rie, H. E. *et al.* (1964) Tutoring and ventilation, *Clinical Paed.* 3, 581–586.
13. The Tunbridge Wells Study Group (1973) Non-accidental injuries to children, in *Special Education*, Spastics Society Publications, London and *Br. Med. J.* 4, 96.

14. Newcastle-upon-Tyne Working Party (1973) Non-accidental injury to children: a guide on management, *Br. med. J.* **4**, 656–660.
15. Helfer, R. E. and Kempe, C. H. (1968) *The Battered Child,* University of Chicago Press, Chicago.
16. Smith, S. M. *et al.* 1973) Parents of battered babies: A controlled study, *Br. med. J.* **4**, 388–391.
17. Skinner, A. (1969) *Battered Children,* Battersea Society for the Prevention of Cruelty to Children, London.
18. MacCarthy, D. and Booth, E. M. (1970) Parental rejection and stunting of growth, *J. Psychosom. Res.* **14**, 259–265.
*19. Joseph, Sir Keith (1973) Communication to Association of Directors of Social Services.
*20. Davie, R. *et al.* (1972) *From Birth to Seven,* Longmans, in association with the National Children's Bureau, London.
21. Crellin, E. *et al.* (1971) *Born Illegitimate,* National Foundation for Educational Research, Slough.
*22. West, D. J. (1967) *The Young Offender,* Pelican Original, Penguin Books, Harmondsworth.
23. Sears, R. R. *et al.* (1957) *Patterns of Child Rearing,* Row, Peterson & Co. Evanston.
24. Newson, J. and Newson, E. (1963) *Infant Care in an Urban Community,* Allen & Unwin and Penguin Books, Harmondsworth, London.
25. Newson, J. and Newson, E. (1968) *Four Years in an Urban Community,* Allen & Unwin, London.
26. *Children and their Primary Schools* (1967) (The Plowden Report), H.M.S.O., London.
27. Halsey, A. (1972) *Educational Priority, H.M.S.O., London.*
28. *Douglas, J. W. B. (1964) The Home and the School,* MacGibbon & Kee, London.
29. Ryan, W. (1971) *Blaming the Victim,* Pantheon, New York.
30. Boxall, M., and Gorell-Barnes, G. (1973) *The Potential for Growth.* Proceedings of NAMH Interclinic Conference, London.
31. Boxall, M. (1973) *Multiple Deprivation: An Experiment in Nurture,* Occasional Paper 2, Division of Educational and Child Psychology of the British Psychological Society, London.
   Gorell-Barnes, G. (1973) Working with the family group, *Social Work Today* **4**, 3, 65–70.

# CHAPTER 4

## *Special Circumstances*

Stressful circumstances and traumatic events must be seen in the light of the total situation in which the child finds himself. For it is not so much the event itself but how the child perceives it which determines the effect it will have on him. Some 'traumatic events' such as birth of a sibling or a separation are so well known that they may be presented by a parent or taken as causative by the doctor whereas some apparently insignificant happening such as the loss of a transitional object at a sensitive stage of development may be more important.

Robert, an intelligent 7-year-old, was an only child who had recently become clinging, refusing to have his mother out of his sight and reluctant to go to school. He had regressed, was soiling, calling himself 'toddler' and wanting to climb into mother's bed. Mother related these symptoms to father's absence on a business trip, since on his return the three of them went on a short holiday during which Robert began to cry and cling to his mother. When she was asked about previous dependency she recalled that Robert had always carried with him a limbless teddy which he would not allow mother to wash or clean in any way. Mother became obsessed with what she called 'that stinking object' and determined to get rid of it. She saw her opportunity when they stopped for a picnic lunch *en route* for the holiday resort. While Robert went for a short walk with his father she threw it into the deepest part of a thorn hedge so there would be no chance of retrieving it when Robert became upset when he failed to find it in the car as they continued their journey. She had completely forgotten this incident.

Some of the situations described in this sector are highly emotive, and I would ask the reader to consider why it is that people judge different aspects of behaviour stemming from the same cause so variously, and why in some instances it is not found possible to look beneath the behaviour to the dynamics.

## A. Overprotection

Levy([1]) has described four signs of overprotection; excessive contact, prevention of independence, lack or excess of maternal control, and infantilism of the child. It is often thought that behind overprotection lies rejection, and indeed these mothers have also known the effect of hunger in their own childhoods plus household cares and responsibilities, and later thwarting of their ambitions by their own parents who remain much in the picture. Marital maladjustment and prolonged anticipation before a child is born are common. These mothers tend to prolong breast feeding and have difficulty in weaning and distancing, feeling that they must be always available. During the 'holding' phase overprotection can do little harm, but it impedes individuation.

Among these mothers one may find over-indulgent mothers who are said to be the masochistic slaves of their child who reigns supreme in the household.

### Authoritarian and rigid parents

These parents (though less obviously) are nevertheless a menace to their child's development. They have been rigidly brought up themselves and see their children as possessions and extensions of themselves, to be moulded to some ideal standard, to some long-term plan which has no regard for the needs of the children. Authority restrictions and punitive measures are used to prevent untoward and dreaded developments especially in the sexual or aggressive fields. Such parents are often 'perfectionistic'. From these families we see children who 'out of the blue' go out and commit some antisocial act, such as Clive, a 13-year-old grammar-school boy, who went off one Saturday afternoon and did several hundreds of pounds worth of damage to a municipal building. Mother's comment was that 'everything would have been all right if he had gone swimming with his older brother as usual'.

### B. Reaction to Having a Damaged Child; Maternal Perplexity

Some aspects of this have been discussed in Chapter 1. Here I want to emphasise how common is the fear of having an abnormal or damaged child, and the first question after delivery is often 'Is it normal?'. The heightened sensitivity of the puerperal mother may cause her to pick up minor degrees of impairment not obvious to others which hinders her rapport with her infant and prevents positive feedback. Reassurance given in answer to her anxious questioning leaves her feeling isolated and inadequate. Mothers of children with minor degrees of mental retardation or autism claim that from the earliest days there was something different about 'this child'. Where the abnormality is more severe the fact that the mother has to hand over the child for a time also leaves her feeling ineffectual.

The infant grows up in an atmosphere not so much of coldness but of anxiety, perplexity and fear.

The term maternal perplexity has been used to describe young, immature or emotionally disturbed mothers who, faced with some abnormality in their child or some minor problem, are not able to 'grow into' their role as mothers, but instead regress to a stage of helplessness. The child responding to this and to the alienation she senses in her mother behaves in an· increasingly uncontrolled or bizarre fashion.

Andrea was a 4-year-old girl who had shown some autistic behaviour since the age of 2. Her mother who had had emotional problems, denied that there was anything wrong with the girl, yet became extremely upset when she showed abnormal behaviour especially in public. Andrea was at her most abnormal when with her mother, but away from her in the company of other members of the family or at nursery school her behaviour was much more normal.

Fortunately handicapped children have two parents, and the kind of care one is able to give may offset the lack or excess of care given by the other, or one parent may be able to provide at one stage while the other may take over later on. Care may be overdone or smothering, or casual and unpredictable; always there is ambivalence, especially as the child grows older and the problems greater. The parents of 'Jo Egg'[2] were ordinary conscientious parents who wanted to do their best for their severely subnormal physically handicapped girl, yet the stress built up to such a point that hostile feelings developed and became overt.

## C. The Sexually Victimised Child*

Children involved in sexual approaches and assaults are not always the innocent 'victims' society and·their parents like to imagine. Child psychiatrists see many young children who are 'at risk' in regard to such offences,

*See also Gibbens and Prince[3], Schultz *et al.*[4].

and many child 'victims' consciously or unconsciously seek to allow affectionate behaviour and consent to the offence or offer little resistance. In many cases the 'attacker' is known to the 'victim' and violence is not employed. In general these sexual assaults do not have an unsettling effect on the child who does not perceive the event at the time as traumatic. Emotional upset may occur secondary to the reaction of panic and fright on the part of parents and society and to the questioning and cross-questioning in and out of court. There seems to be a need for society to indict and punish the offender, and for parents to prove that they are good and conscientious people, and that their child did not in any way invite the assault.

The first duty of the child psychiatrist, as always, is to his patient the child, to help her individually and also to assist the parents to minimise the trauma of the event.

## D. 'Normal' Family Hazards

We have looked at hospitalisation of the child, one effect of which is the limited separation from his parents, and at other situations depriving the child particularly of maternal love. Absence of the father either because his working hours are such that he rarely sees his children or over longer periods will have an effect depending on the stage of development which the child has reached. It is rather like a bereavement and there is a need for the mother to keep the father alive for the child so that on his return there is a warm place for him, so that development of the child may proceed.

Birth of a sibling is an event that tests the young child's success in freeing himself from the need to possess his mother. If he is still a baby, if he has been the only one for a number of years, or was born after a long interval he is unlikely to have achieved this success, and will react by jealousy. He may show this openly even expressing a wish to murder the baby (one toddler pushed the baby out of his pram and got in himself) or may deny it and show extra affection towards him, or he may regress. He may become aggressive to his mother, blaming her for producing a rival. A child's relationship with his siblings sets a pattern for his relationships with other children and with his peers in later life.

Many situations in a family such as unemployment or illness of the father, financial crises, or mother having an operation may be too much for the precarious adjustment of children who are insecure, overdependent or guilt-ridden and they may develop a school refusal or a phobia.

## E. Bereavement

In general a child's attitude to the death of a parent will depend on his age (very young children do not seem aware of the meaning of death) and the way in which deaths of pets, friends or relatives have been dealt with (Anthony ([5])). Often the child is 'shielded' from the knowledge and the same procedure may be followed when a parent dies. The child may even be told that the parent is still in hospital or has gone away; he may not be taken to the hospital nor ever see the grave. The surviving parent may try to hide his distress from the child, yet his grief or guilt is likely to dominate the household. The most adverse effects occur when there has been marital disharmony prior to the death, the child retaining an image of a bad parent or blaming himself. Overtly he may adopt a callous attitude.

In such a situation John, whose father was killed in a road accident near his village, was asking everyone at school if they had seen the photograph of the accident in the newspaper. The sensitive headmaster found this 'shocking'. When there is a death in a family although there is a general feeling of sympathy there is often in addition an embarrassed turning away which feeds into the denial which the family may be showing. When a much-loved partner dies his image can be kept alive in a positive way, and then it may be possible for the surviving parent and the children to share their mourning (Marris([6]); Rutter([7])).

When the mother dies the family often breaks up; when the father dies the family becomes impoverished both financially and emotionally.

## F. Broken and One-parent Homes, Illegitimacy, Separation, Divorce

Again these situations may indicate personality disorders or inadequacies often carried from one generation to the next (Schlesinger([8])). The practical result of illegitimacy may be that the child(ren) is taken into care or brought up by grandparents, and the emotional one that they are left with the picture of a 'bad' parent. Eunice brought up by paternal grandmother (father visited occasionally) was told that her mother was a prostitute, that she stole and lied and lived with black men. One day when walking in the street with her grandmother they saw a drunken woman reeling out of a pub 'That was your mother' said the grandmother scathingly.

One parent (usually mother and child) families may have problems which are financial, medical, and emotional (the lack of a spouse and the lack of a parent). Medical aspects of illegitimacy have been considered earlier (Chapter 3).

The effect on the child of separation and divorce will depend on the age of the child and the way in which the parents are able to relate to one another and deal with such questions as access. Most damaging is where the child is used in a tug-of-war between the parents.

## G. Infertility, Adoption

The special situation presented by adoption starts with the problem of infertility, the reason why the couple have been unable to conceive. Where lies the blame? On the husband, the wife or some incompatability between them? Since both husband and wife are on occasion able to conceive with another partner or even with one another (especially after adopting a child) it appears that more than physical reasons enter into infertility.

The effect is usually hardest on the woman, who feels incomplete, who is more often reminded of parenthood by seeing fulfilled mothers and has fewer outside compensations.

Yerma, who is infertile, speaks to her pregnant friend Maria of the need of women for children. 'Every woman has blood enough for four or five children and when she does not have them they turn to poison within her, as has happened with me.'* 'Artificial insemination' may resolve the problem for some women, but unless the husband is the donor it may increase his difficulty.

Long anticipation of conception or adoption is likely to cause the parents to focus too closely on the child. Adoptive parents often feel less secure than natural parents since they carry a burden of responsibility for the child they have 'chosen', whereas the child carries the weight of having been chosen. One child burst out 'I wish you hadn't chosen me'.

Adoptive parents feel a need to take an active role in the child's development as though to ensure that things 'go right'. They readily become panicky, either blaming themselves or projecting the blame onto the child or the real parents. (Others, including doctors and teachers, may consolidate this by saying 'Well after all he is adopted'.) It is hard to decide when and how to word the telling of the child. Telling early may be advisable so that the child is not told by anyone else, but the phrases 'we adopted you' or 'we chose you' or 'you grew in another mummy's tummy' may mean little to the very

*From *Boda Yerma Sangre*, F. Garcia Lorca(9).

young child or may start off phantasies. It is essential to talk with the child from time to time to see how he is getting along with his adopted state.

Both adoptive parents and adopted child are fearful of rejection, and find it hard to accept the ambivalence in the relationship. It is natural that the child should show curiosity about his own parents and have phantasies that they were wholly good and loving or rich and powerful especially when things go wrong. He may cry 'You are not my mother' or (particularly in adolescence) wish to seek his real parents. The child, having been rejected by his own parents, will readily fear a second rejection especially where natural siblings are born or in a setting of marital disharmony.

Helen, an only adopted child, began stealing and running away from home when her adopted parents separated. She became violent towards her adoptive mother who blamed her for the breakup of the marriage (see McWhinnie[10,11], Pringle[12]).


## H. Fostering*

Parents who adopt usually do so in order to have a child to bring up as their own 'as long as they all shall live'; most often to fill a gap, since they are not able to have children (or more children) of their own, but some for altruistic reasons.

The motivation of foster parents is more varied. It may sometimes be a means of making money (though not very much), quite often by doing something which the foster mother (in particular) is good at (i.e. looking after children). Such parents do not foster because they need the money, but they need the money in order to be able to foster, and Adamson (1973) has shown that these foster parents may be among the best.

Short-term fostering is usually done by those who wish to offer a service without becoming emotionally involved with the children, whatever age they may be, perhaps because they have a family of their own. Parents who foster after their own children are grown up may also wish to avoid over-involvement, but in some cases the real wish is to have a young child or even a baby still in the family.

When couples take on a 'family' of foster children (not of course necessarily from the same family) the emotional attachment to the children tends to be diluted by the fact of the numbers.

*See George[13], Ballance[14].

Sometimes a short-term fostering becomes long-term on account of circumstances; the original fostering may have been arranged because of a special appeal inherent in the situation, which in turn makes a special tie between the child and the foster parents. When the planned return to the natural parents is not possible the fostering continues.

Where long-term fostering of a single child is arranged, particularly when the parents have no children of their own, the situation may be very close to adoption, and one may wonder why adoption was not sought. In some cases it may have been, but there may have been some doubt about the suitability of the parents, or fostering with a view to adoption may be arranged in the hope that the natural parents will eventually agree. Or there may have been some doubt about the child, and a period during which the child's growth and development may be observed is required. When the opportunity to adopt occurs the fosterparents may delay.

Some couples may wish to have a child to call their own, but are unable to adopt for financial reasons. Sometimes there is an inexplicable holding back, the couple are always about to 'apply to adopt him' but they never do. When they have made promises to their foster child this is very upsetting for him. The hardest case is where the hope of adoption is always just around the corner but each time the natural parent refuses at the last minute.

## Short-term fostering

This is usually arranged because of some natural or unnatural emergency in the family, or, in the case of babies, prior to adoption.

The natural parents may worry about how their child will be cared for, and the Robertson's films have demonstrated how important it is for the child to get to know the foster mother and the foster home prior to his arrival there, and to be able to bring some part of his own home with him, and to keep it alive as far as is possible. On the other hand when the foster home is clearly doing a better job than the real home, it may underline the inadequacy of the natural parents, and even turn them against the child.

## Long-term fostering

If the child is out of babyhood, he needs to be introduced gradually to the foster home, and it is important to assess when he is ready to make the final move into his new home.

There are three parties to be considered in the fostering situation, the child, the foster parents, and the natural parents.

Where the natural parents (or parent) are still active in the situation or where the child has potent memories of a parent, there may be a conflict of loyalties, or even confusion about 'which Mummy to love'. If the parent turns up from time to time, and especially if she talks of having the child back the situation is very tense and uneasy. When the parent is almost forgotten, a card or small present may arrive at Christmas.

Often the child feels he belongs wholly to the foster parents, just as an adopted child may, and should the real parents claim their rights a tragic situation may arise. Or the foster child may settle happily until adolescence, when the 'normal' adolescent protest, rejection and search for identity, may rock the foster home and the foster parents. Children who have been deprived or who come from very disturbed backgrounds may become very stormy during adolescence. The need to trace parents and have knowledge of their antecedents is as strong in foster children as in adopted children.

Yet foster parents have persistent problems which adoptive parents do not know; the awareness that the child may be 'taken back', but also the need, if they are to be truly generous and loving to him, to help him to see and imagine himself as part of his original family. If they cannot do this they are failing to accept him wholly. Vulnerable foster parents may seek to deny that other family, may refuse to give the foster child information, or letters which are sent, may insist on a change of name to their name and so on.

The natural parents may have ambivalent feelings about letting their child go to foster parents, and may genuinely believe that they will 'have him back' one day. Mothers particularly may find visits to the foster home upsetting, and the better it is the worse she may feel. She may shower the child with gifts and promises, or alternatively fail to turn up, having got cold feet at the last minute. The foster mother can help the natural mother if she understands and accepts these feelings and actions.

The social worker is in the middle, and in order to serve the needs of the child she must understand the problems of both sets of parents. To the foster mother she may be the reminder of the precariousness of the situation; that her care is under scrutiny, that the child could be taken back. (This could be done by the natural parents, but also by the Social Service Department). The foster mother may resent the interest the social worker takes in the child, feeling that this is her prerogative. (Indeed in some instances when the social worker takes over tasks a natural parent would expect to do, such as taking the child to a clinic or to a boarding school, she, the foster mother, may well be right.)

How far it is possible for the social worker to help the foster parents to see the foster child through his identity and other crises, and how far she needs to deal directly with him is a moot point, but where she does choose the latter course the feelings of exclusion which the foster parents feel must be understood. How the child sees the foster parents will be affected by how the social worker plays her part, as will his relationship to the social worker herself. Although the latter may be able to play the role of 'confidant' for the adolescent, it must be remembered that this may be more threatening to the foster parents than if an outsider or family friend does it.

The social worker may remind the real parent of her failures and guilt, or she may see her as a helpful person who facilitates her contacts with her child and with the foster parents.

The social worker has a difficult part to play in this triangular situation which may last the whole of the child's young life.

## I. Step Parents

Here the situation is complex and taxing. A stepmother, for example, has to accept and care for a child(ren) not her own and adapt to a new husband while the child who has lost one mother has to accept partially at least a replacement and see that person in a close relationship with the father. When the stepmother brings children of her own into the family, loyalties and rivalries between the sibs and stepsibs add to the complications as when the absent parents remain active in the situation.

Donald, aged 8, developed encopresis following his father's remarriage. His mother had died when he was 3 from a recurrence of cancer. Donald (and probably father) blamed himself for her death. He was brought up by maternal grandparents who strove to keep his mother's memory alive. Father remarried when Donald was 7 and they went to live 100 miles away. Donald's stepmother had two children from her previous marriage, the younger girl she brought with her, the boy the same age as Donald remained with his father.

The general attitude towards illegitimacy, separation and divorce, infertility adoption and step-parenthood is mixed indeed but there is probably a gradual increase in sympathy as we go along this list. Yet overt sympathy may mask latent hostility which is shown by tactless remarks made to parents who are infertile or who have adopted a child.

## Bibliography and Further Reading

Items marked * are particularly important sources. Unnumbered references provide alternative sources to the reference quoted immediately above.

*1.    Levy, D. M. (1943) *Maternal Overprotection,* Columbia Press, New York.
2.    Nicholls, P. (1967) A Day in the Death of Jo Egg, Faber. London.
3.    Gibbens, T. C. N. and Prince, J. (1963) *Child Victims of Sex Offences,* Institute for the Study and Treatment of Delinquency (ISTD) Publications, London.
4.    Schultz, L. *et al.* (1972) Psychotherapeutic and legal approaches to the sexually victimised child, *Int. J. Child Psychother,* 1, 115–128.
5.    Anthony, S. (1940) *The Child's Discovery of Death,* Kegan Paul, Trench, Trubner Co., London.
6.    Marris, P. (1958) *Widows and their Families,* Routledge & Kegan Paul, London.
7.    Rutter, M. (1966) *Children of Sick Parents,* Maudsley Monograph No. 16, Oxford University Press, London.
*8.    Schlesinger, P. (1969) *The One Parent Family.* Toronto University Press, Toronto.
9.    Garcia Lorca, F. *Boda Yerma Sangre.*
10.    McWhinnie, A. (1973) Adoption, in *Services for Children and their Families* (ed. Stroud, J.), Pergamon Press, Oxford.
11.    McWhinnie, A. (1967) *Adopted Children: How They Grow Up,* Routledge & Kegan Paul, London.
     McWhinnie, A. (1973) Adoption, in *Services for Children and their Families,* (ed. Stroud, J.). Pergamon Press, Oxford.
*12.    Pringle, M. K. (1967) *Adoption Facts and Fallacies,* Longmans, London.
*    Gray, E. and Blunden, R. (1971) *A Survey of Adoption in Great Britain,* H.M.S.O., London.
13.    George, V. (1970) *Foster Care,* Routledge & Kegan Paul, London.
     Raynor, L. (1970) *Adoption of Non-White Children,* Allen & Unwin, London.
*    Stroud, J. (ed.) (1973) *Services for Children and their Families,* Pergamon Press, Oxford.
14.    Ballance, G. (1973) Fostering, in *Services for Children and their Families* (ed. Stroud, J.), Pergamon Press, Oxford.
*    Wolff, S. (1969) *Children under Stress,* Allen Lane, The Penguin Press, London.

## CHAPTER 5

# Family Factors

The reader may well say 'We have been thinking about the family all this time'. Aspects of role playing and family living have received extra attention from researchers into family pathology and from family therapists, and it is the views of some of these workers which will be highlighted in this section and again in the section on family therapy.

## A. Mother and Father

The parents have been called by Satir([1]) 'the architects of the family'. It is they who serve as models for the children in sex dominance, aggression and attitudes towards work and authority. Satir traces the way in which the grandparents modelled for the parents (and may still) just as the parents are being models for the child. This kind of emphasis immediately puts the father in the forefront of the picture along with the mother. For some time there have been attempts to modify the popular idealisation of the mother-child dyad, but it was an essay of T. Main([2]) which set out to shatter the complacency. First he looked at the polarisation between the 'good' and 'bad' ('Madonna' and 'Witch') mothers. He demonstrated the pathology behind the behaviour of some 'Madonnas' (more mothers than wives) whose preoccupation with their infant enables them to retreat from their infantile sexual problems and exclude the father from the parenting and marital situations. More obvious was the pathology of the 'Witch' mother (more wife than mother) who might turn completely from husband and child, even denying that the infant is hers, and handing him over to others. Secondly, he deplored the use of the names 'Mother, Father, Child' rather than 'Wife, Husband, Child' and the separation of the wifely from the maternal role, with a stereotype of the woman considered solely in her maternal role of devotion to her one infant and ignoring her feminine and wifely roles. Women in whom these aspects are strong may feel guilty and inadequate as mothers, and may even become depressed. They may allow themselves to be taken care of in hospital and willingly hand over the care of their infant in order to keep him safe, but Main considers that it is not always necessary or wise to take from these mothers the care of their infants. Help given then and afterwards (both to mothers identified as 'patients' and those 'at risk' in maternity wards) may prevent long-term failures of parenting such as we have seen in the case of mothers who cannot keep a safe home.

The father's role in supporting the mother-child 'unity' and in compensating for lacks can be clearly perceived, but he too needs to be seen as the partner of his wife, which relationship predates that of father to his child.

Ideally there should be in the relationship of husband and wife a complementarity in that together there is a fit and completeness, and a reciprocity in that there is movement and mutuality between them. These aspects have been stressed by both Satir([1]) and Ackerman.([3]).

## B. Parenthood

What happens when these aspects are lacking can be seen when Jack M. and Jill M. husband and wife, become a family on the arrival of their first child. There is immediately a change of emphasis from their mutual needs to the needs and rearing of children, with the addition of new responsibilities. This puts a strain on a marriage which is precarious on account of the youth and immaturity of the parents. How in fact can they begin to be parents when they have unresolved childish needs themselves? Even where the couple have looked forward to the arrival of the child as a sharing process which will enhance their relationship, each may also be looking for personal satisfaction through the child. They may both still be affected by the interaction of their own parents and the partners may be looking for the same interaction (or its opposite) in each other. If the role is not filled the spouse may look for it or for lost aspects of his own personality or missed satisfactions in the child.

Such parents who think they live for the child, or who live through the child or have the child live for them; or who find unacceptable aspects of parents, spouse or in-laws appearing in a child may have difficulties in parenting which may account, at least in part, for prejudicial scapegoating of one child in the family. At the time of marriage the partners may have unrealistic hopes of having their needs met (at last) and when disappointed may turn to the children for satisfaction. Polarisation between the two parents, or between one parent and a child or between a parent and his own parent may result. Or again there may be a clash between mothering (or indeed fathering) in or outside the home.

Mr and Mrs Jones had met at work. She was a factory hand and he, with an incompleted degree in engineering behind him, a floor manager. Mrs J. who had career ambitions which she had never even started to develop, saw herself sharing by proxy in Mr J's work and leisure activities almost as a partner, while he saw her as taking an intelligent interest in his work, but by way of listening to him in awed wonderment while she fed their baby at the breast. Yet the couple had never discussed 'having kids' which she did not want. She claimed that her two children were 'unplanned' but he did not agree, since they had 'never taken precautions'. Mrs J spoke almost proudly of the fact that she 'rejected' the little girls from the start along with all aspects of domestic 'drudgery'. She took a marked interest in Mr J's work even to expecting to be able to choose his jobs for him, and took on work outside the home herself but let the house become what an infuriated Mr J. called 'a tip'.

It is easy to see that whatever the origins of such attitudes may have been neither had complementarity nor reciprocity in their relationship and the elder girl particularly, born at a time of greatest frustration and minimum accommodation had become seriously disturbed.

Some fathers (less trapped by economic circumstances than Mr J.) may engage in excessive extroverted activity outside the home either in business, social or sporting activities. Such fathers may find difficulty in combining fatherly or even husbandly roles with these other masculine roles. If they are not helped by emotional feedback from the wife-mother, the children, following her lead may become estranged from their father regarding him as an interloper or a visitor. A wife in this situation where the husband is frequently absent, may, in spite of protestations to the contrary, gain some satisfaction from the aversion or neglect shown by the children to the father, especially as this keeps them for her.

## C. Extended Family

Nuclear families are part of a larger group or even of a clan, members of which influence the family for good or ill, first and foremost the grandparents. The active presence of grandparents on one or both sides of the family may enhance or diminish family bonds. Where the spouses have been able to free themselves from excessive emotional ties to their own parents and this has been well accepted, the latter are able to offer a truly supportive role to the family. Owing to their relative distance from responsibility they can provide a caring non-critical relationship to the child, leaving to its parents their roles in regard to decisions and discipline. A certain amount of child spoiling can be accepted by parents who do not feel they have gone short in affection and attention themselves, and the help given by grandparents may afford them the opportunity of being a 'couple' again.

It is unfortunate therefore that tensions often arise, especially where a dominant parent is seen to be exercising that same dominance over a new generation or where there is favouritism, particularly if that recreates a situation in the parent's own childhood. Conflicting feelings of affection, irritation and guilt may in any case plague relationships with grandparents and where the parents themselves do not agree polarisation may result either between a particular grandchild and a particular grandparent, or between a grandparent and one of the spouses.

Thus it appears that ability to relate with and use the extended family, and particularly grandparents, is a measure of a healthy functioning family, and N. Bell[4] has suggested that disturbed families can be distinguished from well families by their patterns of relationships with extended families, since extended families serve as screens for the projection of conflicts, and also compete for scarce resources (mainly material goods and affection). In many disturbed families the generation boundaries are blurred since members of the different generations all make excessive demands, and extended kin tend to become involved in family conflicts. A particular member of the extended family may assume paramount importance in decision-making in the family. This could be any member, usually but not necessarily older than the parents, and possibly a relation by marriage and this person has been named by Bowen[5] 'Head of the Clan'.

We have been thinking about family boundaries and have seen that families are systems which are not closed. It seems appropriate to point to the broader systems involving culture and community, which may also function to stimulate conflicts, or to correct or contain them.

Kluckhohn[6] has studied societal and cultural effects on the whole family field, Bowen[5] examined the boundaries or distancing between individual family members and the boundary of the whole family system and J. G. Miller[7] has followed the broader approach in his study of Living Systems.

## D. The Children

It seems most unlikely that parent's frequent claim 'We treat them all alike' can be substantiated; rather, each child has a unique experience in family life; because of position in regard to birth order, sex, gap between next oldest and next youngest, the family situation at the time of conception and birth, and finally factors inherent in the child. Two research studies are quoted, one on parental attitudes with a fairly wide base, and one on sibling constellations with a narrower one.

The Fels Research Institute of Ohio State University examined parental attitudes to first and second children, and also subsequent children, and found that behaviour to the first as contrasted to the second child, is less warm emotionally and more restrictive and coercive, especially during the pre-school years. This difference appeared also, although less distinctly between second and third children. There is less parent-child interaction as the first child gets older, but attitudes change less towards later-born children. The factor most affecting behaviour of parents is the age difference between siblings, and a somewhat surprising finding is that closely spaced children are on the whole more advantageously treated than widely spaced children. Overall, parents tend to be self-consistent in their methods of handling their children (Lasko[8]).

Schmuck[9] quotes Adler's[10] classical speculations about birth order in his carefully circumscribed study of conformity in female college students in relation to birth order and sex of sibling in two-child families. He found that sex of sibling was the important variable and that girls with a sister were more rebellious than girls with a brother.

### Methods of Child rearing

The findings of Brody and Robertson have already been mentioned in Part 1. Their suggestion that the way the mother feels about the feeding method selected greatly affects the way the infant perceives the situation, is borne out by a retrospective study on self-evaluation in normal children by Coopersmith[25]. He found that parental satisfaction with the method chosen for feeding, weaning, toilet training, etc. and the consistency and firmness with which it was used correlated with the development of high self-esteem in the child.

### E. Communication within the Family

Great interest has been taken in the ways in which a family communicates. Satir in fact lays the whole blame for 'family trouble' on failure of communication stemming from the marital couple and pervading the whole family. A particular child (who later becomes the 'identified patient') is for some reason particularly vulnerable and grows up in an environment where communication between his parents confuses him in various ways. For example the mother may talk about the husband in one way but treat him in another (and expect the child to treat the father in a different way from the way she does). Nothing ever gets brought out into the open, secrets kept within the family or away from a particular family member feed into the feeling that the truth could be damaging and cause the family to fall apart. Messages as well as being confusing to the child are also devaluing. In this kind of a family differences cannot be accepted, but instead there is a need for sameness as though to protect the family from dissolution. Family members often play roles which are not congruous with their position in the family or with what they say about themselves.

A family may reveal itself by its method of taking decisions. Decision may be by consensus with all members holding the same view, or by accommodation; some members compromising, or by imposition by one or more powerful figures. The most effective from a long-term point of view seems to be a co-operative system with one person (not necessarily always the same one) who has the ability to evaluate conflicting ideas and family goals acting as co-ordinator.

### F. Growth Needs of the Family

We have seen that for healthy emotional growth the child requires to have his phase-bound needs met, and for his environment to facilitate his surmounting of the developmental hurdles. V. Satir has summarised growth needs within the family. The child needs to find a role for himself which is not dependent on what his parents hope to find in him, and a value given for himself which is not solely dependent on what he may achieve. He needs to feel some status and dignity, although he is a child among adults much more powerful than he, and to achieve a balance between dependence and independence within his family. He needs to have his aggressive and sexual strivings recognised without hostility, and to be able to communicate negative as well as positive feelings towards his parents without losing their love, and also to accept their ambivalent feelings towards himself. In 'troubled families' we need to ask: who labelled what behaviour as a symptom, and what does the symptom say about discrepancies between the rules of the family and the growth needs of the individuals in it? The obverse of this is, what does the symptom say about trouble, pain or confusion in the rest of the family? (Ackerman([11])).

Both Satir and Bowen point to lack of recognition of uniqueness and separateness, and ability of family members to distance themselves, in families where there is a 'symptom bearer'.

*Strengths in the Family, 'homeostasis'*

Ackerman([12]) in particular has been interested in strengths in the collective family, and in 'restitution processes'. A family by working together may find means of coping with stress from without and conflicts from within. A problem may be lessened by strengthening the bonds of love, by seeking a shared solution, by a change in family roles or a shift in alignment; or even by a change in the external environment or by the temporary elimination of one family member and the introduction of another.

Some families actually seem to improve under stress. Anthony([13]) studied family functioning before and after illness of family members (mental and physical) and found that in some 'profiles' the family reached a higher level of organisation after than before the illness.

The concept of 'homeostasis' (dynamic equilibrium or steady state) has been used to describe the way in which an organism in face of stress leading to strain seeks to adjust itself and return to the 'steady state'. The concept has also been used to describe the developing individual, and Ackerman([14]) in particular has used the term 'family homeostasis' to describe a situation where if members of a family continue to live together there develops a kind of self-corrective process to make this continued association possible, even in the face of continuing conflicts. Ackerman considers that each family has its own homeostat suited to it, with its own dynamics and rules which it uses to govern behaviour and communication. Time and habit serve to strengthen the system which may be favourable or unfavourable for the growth of family members.

## G. The Functioning Family

Just as we may have a well- or ill-functioning marital dyad or nursing couple, so we may have a well- or ill-functioning family of which the smallest number is the triad or mother, father, child. Is it possible to have a model of a family which functions well? Most models would present a tall order for many of the families we come across in our work but will serve to summarise this section.

Lidz looks at roles, and suggests that the need is for an effective parental coalition with appropriate sharing of roles affording roles for the children to follow, and with the generation boundaries maintained so that the children do not have to satisfy the unmet needs of the parents.

This view is close to Satir, who also stresses communication of family members with one another and with the outside world.

Ackerman looks to smooth functioning, shown by multiple accommodation methods which are repeatedly evaluated, to flexibility and to ability to act in concert. The greatest needs are for stability and identity, and he considers that a family which has little confidence in its identity may have identity foisted on it from outside. Though the family homeostat may be threatened in many ways he has great hope for family problem-solving.

Skynner is particularly interested in the levels of personal integration within the family and the ways in which a given family situation may deprive some of its members of opportunities to meet and master some crucial developmental stage.

## H. Prejudicial Scapegoating

Skynner([15]) and Ackerman([14]) have described how in 'neurotic' families the unresolved childhood conflicts of one or both parents are repeatedly enacted. The child is given a role which in some way expresses or satisfies the parent's immaturity, inadequacy or neurotic conflict. Ackerman describes how parental pathology may be distributed among the children in the family so that one child becomes aggressive while another becomes timid and submissive. Ackerman describes prejudicial scapegoating (as seen in the case of Kevin) whereby one family member is picked out often from birth because of some difference he shows which is felt to be a menace to family continuity. A 'game' develops with victim and persecutor, often with changing alignments or even multiple scapegoating, and a 'family healer' may be involved. The victim may escape, be replaced by another family member or become emotionally ill. Sometimes the family seems to be held together by the game, at others it may be divisive.

In other cases the child acts out the parent's sexual or aggressive anti-authority feelings, or where parenthood has upset a precarious balance there may be simply irritability and constant picking on the child.

Close to the idea of scapegoating is the 'family myth' as described by A. Ferreira[16]. The myth which may involve the parents, one parent or one child is to the relationship or to the family 'what the defence is to the individual', protecting the system against the threat of disintegration. The myth could be the strength of illness or instability of an individual member, and the family cling to this especially when stability is threatened.

## I. Cross-cultural Studies

As a check and perhaps a corrective in regard to the emphasis placed on the family and particularly the mother in the development of the young child, we can look to cultures who rear their children differently from us. Mead[17] from her cross-cultural studies has condemned the over-emphasis on the psychological tie between the infant and his biological mother, considering that adjustment is best if the child is cared for by many warm and friendly people. More relevant are studies of societies in which the young children are reared apart from their natural parents. An obvious example is Kibbutzism in Israel (see Irvine[18]).

The general pattern is that although children from birth live in children's homes the natural mother participates a great deal in early infant care. She does not work during the first 6 weeks, and during this time and up to 9 months (when she is back to full-time work) she feeds her baby and cares for him, the care being gradually taken over by his particular nurse. Mother and father continue to visit and in many cases the grandmother is active in providing play and stimulation for the child. At 1 year the infant moves to a toddler house with the group of infants he has been with where he remains with a new nurse to care for him and train him, but with the parents and other members of the family visiting in the evenings. At 4 or sometimes at 7 several houses are combined to form a school and one or more teachers are introduced.

In each Kibbutz the pattern is the same for all the children, thus the unfavourable effect when only some mothers work, or where a mother works spasmodically and the child has to get used to both a working and a non-working mother is avoided.

A number of workers have studied Kibbutz children at various ages, and also Kibbutz-reared adults but clearly found it difficult to decide whether they should study developmental quotients, intellectual achievements or emotional adjustment (Rabin,[19,21]) (Bettleheim,[20] Miller[22]) and Gewirtz[23]).

On the whole Rabin's conclusion was substantiated, i.e. that 'Kibbutz multiple mothering has no long-range deleterious effects upon personality development and character structure', and from Rabin that the kibbutznick was 'healthy, intelligent, generous and shy but warm.' There were indications of some levelling in attainments and similarity in behaviour, but in general Kibbutz-reared children were similar to multiple child families and different from institutionalised children. But Bettleheim did, however, consider that Kibbutz-reared children have problems in their personal relationships and pointed especially to the difficulties which arose in their marriages in relation to intimacy.

## Bibliography and Further Reading

Items marked * are particularly important sources. Unnumbered references provide alternative sources to the reference quoted immediately above.

1. Satir, V. (1964) *Conjoint Family Therapy,* Science and Behaviour Books, Palo Alto.
2. Main, T. (1968) A fragment on mothering, in *Psychosocial Nursing* (ed. Barnes, E.), Social Science Paperbacks, in association with Tavistock Press, London.
*3. Ackerman, N. (1958) *The Psychodynamics of Family Life,* Basic Books, New York.
4. Bell, N. (1962) Extended family relations of disturbed and well families, *Family Process,* 1, 2, 175–193.
5. Bowen, Murray (1972) *Family Interaction* (ed. Framor, J. L.), 183–197.
6. Kluckholm, F. (1958) Variations in the basic values of family systems, *Social Casework* 39, 1/2, 63–72.
7. Miller, J. G. (1965) Living systems, in *Basic Concepts in Behavioural Science,* 10, 337–379.
8. Lasko, J. K. (1954) Parent behaviour toward first and second child, *Genetic Psychology Monographs,* 49, 97–137.
9. Schmuck, R. (1963) Sex of sibling, birth order position and female disposition to conform in two-child families, *Child Dev.* 34, 3, 913–918.
10. Adler, A. (1938) *Social Interest: A Challenge to Mankind,* Faber & Faber, London.
*11. Ackerman, N. (1966) *Treating the Troubled Family,* Basic Books, New York.

*See also Kardiner and Linton[24] for a general description of cultural systems.

*12. Ackerman, N. (1954) Interpersonal disturbances in the family, *Psychiatry* **17**, 359–368.

*13. Anthony, E. J. (1970) The mutative impact of serious mental and physical illness in a parent on family life, in *The Child in his Family* (eds. Anthony, E. J. and Koupernik, C.), Wiley–Interscience, New York.

14. Ackerman, N. (1964) Prejudicial scrapegoating and neutralising forces in the family group, *Int. J. Soc. Psychiat.* (Congress issue), **43**.

15. Skynner, A. C. R. (1967) Diagnosis, consultation and coordination of treatment, in *Papers Given at the 23rd Child Guidance Interclinic Conference*, National Association for Mental Health, London.

16. Ferreira, A. J. (1963) *Family myth and homeostasis Arch. Psychiat.* **9**, 5, 457–463.

17. Mead, M. (1954) Some theoretical considerations of the problem of mother-child separation, *Am. J. Orthopsychiat.* **24**, 471–483.

*18. Irvine, E. (1966) Children in Kibbutzim: thirteen years after, *J. Child Psychol. Psychiat.* **7**, 3/4, 167–178.

19. Rabin, A. I. (1965) *Growing up in the Kibbutz*, Springer, New York.

20. Bettelheim, B. (1969) *The Children of the Dream*, Macmillan, London.

21. Rabin, A. I. (1969) Of dreams and reality; Kibbutz children, *Children*, **16**, 3, 160–162.

*22. Miller, L. (1969) Child-rearing in the Kibbutz, in *Modern Perspectives of International Child Psychiatry* (ed. Howells, J. G.), Oliver & Boyd, Edinburgh.

23. Gewitz, H. B. and Gewitz, J. L. (1969) Caretaking settings, background events and behaviour differences in four Israeli child-rearing environments, in *Determinants of Infant Behaviour* (ed. Foss, B. M.), Methuen, London.

24. Kardiner, A. and Linton, R. (1939) *The Individual and his Society*, Columbia Press, New York.

25. Coopersmith, S. (1967) *The Antecedents of Self Esteem*, Freeman, London.

### PART II

# The Disturbed Child as Patient

*In medical practice – and child psychiatry is one speciality in this field – we think of a child patient as a person who is sick, with various signs and symptoms of illness, and everyone is sympathetic to the child.*

*The child who attends a child psychiatric clinic is in a different position. In a few instances he may appear ill, may tremble, look pale, bite his nails or complain of headache; more often he does not feel ill, and he does not 'complain' of anything. If asked why he has come to the clinic he is often at a loss. 'My mummy brought me', 'Because I've been naughty', 'I can't do my work at school', or perhaps with head hung, 'I wet the bed'.*

*It seems that the person complaining about the child's state is not the child himself but some other person, parent or perhaps school teacher. The complaint may be about behaviour 'signs' or 'symptoms'.*

CHAPTER 6

## Signs and Symptoms of Disturbance

### A. Signs of Disturbance. The Life Style

We will see that these mainly relate to problems of development, and the following are most common.

### 1. Emotional immaturity

This overworked term does describe a characteristic of many disturbed children who show emotional development inappropriate to their chrono-logical age. The child may have failed to mature or he may have advanced and later regressed in the face of difficulties. His total behaviour fits an earlier phase of development. Or the child may have progressed in an average or above average manner in some respects (usually physical and intellectual) with emotional development lagging behind.

William was a 13-year-old boy doing well academically at a traditional grammar school, who had been 'taken away' from a 'progressive' boarding school because it was feared he was getting into 'subversive' company. His family: father a rigid 'army' man, mother emotional and neurotic, younger brother, conforming and immature. William made a demonstrative suicidal attempt (he took 15 aspirins and then phoned the Samaritans for whom his mother worked). He could have passed for 17; tall with long, fair hair, he wore 'trendy' clothes (when out of school uniform) and intellectualised everything in a rather haughty manner. Although he claimed to despise the clinic (imposed on him by his parents whom he also denigrated), he came alone and never missed an appointment. He gradually revealed himself as a 'little boy lost' desperately seeking warmth and care, which, in short supply in his family, mostly went to his younger brother.

## 2. Social difficulties

Related to immaturity, these are very commonly found among children attending the clinic. Failure to get along with the peer group is usual. The child may make, but cannot keep, a friend, he may become the victim of bullying or name-calling, or he may withdraw from social contact with other children, hibernating at home, where he enjoys solitary pursuits or spends time with his parents or other adults (these children often seem like miniature grown-ups). Alternatively the child may relate quite well to older children and adults, or to younger children or children of the opposite sex, enjoying games inappropriate to his age or sex, and further alienating himself from his peers. An interest in team games is unusual, a poor sport, a poor loser, 'he takes his bat home'.

All this throws him back on the home, where feuds with siblings, and irritation of parents, become the rule. At school he is insolent or aggressive towards authority figures, and from being 'a nuisance' he becomes 'unbearable' and finally 'incorrigible'.

## 3. Dissatisfaction

This too seems to belong to a younger age (of omnipotence). Parents say, 'he thinks money grows on trees', 'the grass is always greener on the other side of the fence'. The child is never satisfied, the more he gets the more he wants, things never quite come up to expectation. His attitude to possessions and gifts suggests a deep unease; although so demanding and possessive of what he has (refusing to share with other children) he either destroys expensive gifts or quickly puts them aside.

Graham was a 9-year-old adopted boy under threat of being expelled from a boarding preparatory school. He had a younger non-adopted sister still at home. Mother was pleading with Graham to 'behave' at school. 'I'll buy you that canoe you've always wanted'. Graham flung her away 'Yes, you'd give me the crown jewels if you could' he cried scathingly.

## 4. Intolerance of frustration

The child gives up in the face of the smallest difficulty or sets himself goals he cannot possibly reach. One 5-year-old boy said, 'I want to do something I can't do.' The combination of a high level of aspiration with low tolerance to frustration often leads to outbursts of ungovernable rage (temper tantrums). Or frustration may be the result of excessive pressure put on the child especially in school when he may opt out of the learning situation altogether.

## 5. Facing reality

Most children show great resilience, taking upsets and difficulties in their stride but certain children seem 'vulnerable' or 'fragile' in this respect, and may seek refuge in the excessive use of defence mechanisms. Usually one mechanism is preferred. The parents do not understand. 'He couldn't care less' says his mother, 'I give him a tanning and the next minute he's forgotten it' says Dad. He is impenitent. 'He won't cry for me' sadly from one mother. He looks like becoming a hardened criminal. He is never to blame. 'I didn't do it, they pick on me.'

Other parents accept everything the child tells them and run complaining to the school. Even when they know how difficult the child is they cannot face him with it. Tom's mother received frequent complaints from school and neighbours about his behaviour. 'But I feel so sorry for him' she said. Naturally Tom always ran to her for support.

They may deny that a painful event has occurred. Peter, who had no father, had always been taken to school by his grandfather. When the latter died, mother told Peter that his grandfather had gone to hospital, then that he had gone away. Peter became encopretic and refused to go to school.

Some children evade reality completely escaping into a world of phantasy, others become over-cleanly conforming and moral. Or they may sublimate, engaging excessively in creative sporting or other activities. (No-one is likely to 'complain' of this which may, however, be a sign of disturbance.)

### 6. Learning difficulties

Often present in disturbed children, even when they are not the reason for referral. Concentration may be lacking, the child flitting from one activity to another, or there is an emotional block to learning and knowing, leading especially to reading and other difficulties in communication. More deeply there may be an inhibition of curiosity and experimentation leading to impoverishment of mental functioning and an inability to engage in play and creative activities. Anxiety over relationships and sexual matters is often a factor.

## B. The Symptom

### 1. Symptom as communication

Every symptom whether it be bedwetting, night terrors, stealing or withdrawal is a communication. Overtly a 'cry for help', covertly a communication with a meaning. The meaning is not always the same, stealing for example may have as many different meanings as a physical symptom such as headache, and since the emotional symptom is personal to the child a great deal of detective work may have to be done to discover the meaning.

### 2. Adaptive or maladaptive?

We have seen that the child patient does not see himself as the person who complains of his behaviour does, so his cry for help may not be heard as such, and indeed he may fare worse as a result of his symptom than he did before. In this way a symptom may be seen as maladaptive, yet the same symptom in another context may appear adaptive.

John was 3 when his young sister was born. Previously toilet trained, he began wetting the bed and crawling around on all fours. His mother, recognising his need, arranged to spend several periods of the day alone with him. John was soon back to normal.

Elizabeth was also 3 when her sister was born, and she also began wetting the bed and behaving in a babyish fashion. Her mother found this 'disgusting', told Elizabeth 'You are a big girl now', and left her with the daily help while she went out visiting with the new baby. Elizabeth became a very withdrawn child whose only positive action was to scream loudly from her bed just as her parents were sitting down to their evening meal.

Why does a child continue behaviour which provokes only punishment or rejection? Not only does he do so, but his behaviour becomes more and more outrageous and provocative until some notice, often punitive, is taken. Any attention seems to be better than none. However the attention may 're-inforce' the behaviour and parents and child become locked in a battle, the parents feeling that they must act so the child does not 'get away with it' and the child responding to the challenge.

Rose was a highly intelligent 4-year-old with intellectual parents and a much-indulged brother of 2. Her obsessional mother decided that the little girl should tidy her toys away every evening. Rose refused. On the second occasion mother threatened to throw the toys which were still scattered around the floor into the dustbin. 'Do that' said Rose. Father pleaded with her, 'If only you'd be good for Mummy we wouldn't have to scold you.' Rose still refused. The parents said that if Rose hadn't put her toys away by the time Daddy came home she wouldn't have her usual playtime with him.

Battles continued over the toy situation, but were now extended to mealtimes, bedtimes and every aspect of Rose's life except nursery school where she was a lively easy child. Very occasionally there was a 'good moment' for Rose and her mother 'As though she'd forgotten' Mother remarked showing some insight. Then Daddy would play with her, but he said 'Wouldn't it be lovely if you could be like this every day' and the whole thing started up again.

In some cases of apparently maladaptive behaviour there may be a secondary gain such as aggression directed to an envied sibling or to a figure representing such a sibling, or the child may gain satisfaction from behaviour which hits the parents 'where it hurts most' such as the middle-class child who acts in an antisocial manner.

### 3. Self-rewarding or instrumental

Although most childhood behaviour is instrumental in that it seeks a response (obvious examples are crying or clinging) in some cases the behaviour seems to be an end in itself; examples are thumbsucking, masturbation, nailbiting. These are sometimes known as comfort habits; parents do not usually seek to terminate them unless they are used excessively, are seen to be inappropriate on account of age, or threaten some physical malformation.

### 4. Age-linked symptom

Certain symptoms or groups of symptoms are common at particular stages of childhood. In the very young child, sleep disturbances (difficulty in falling asleep, fitful sleep, early waking) and feeding difficulties (poor appetite, faddiness) but both these and problems over toilet training tend to pass unless the parents over-react. It is noteworthy that these three situations, bedtimes, mealtimes and toilet-times are most likely to form the setting for parent-child confrontations.

From 3 onwards the child may show fears and anxieties, may wake up terrified and insist on bedtime rituals, which may take on an obsessional character. Later true phobic symptoms may develop such as fear of animals or particular objects or noises, but these are so common they can be disregarded unless they increase or become fixed. There is also a danger of recurrence at adolescence. (See Paul, Chapter 2.)

### 5. Attempts at self cure

It will be clear that a symptom as well as having many meanings, may have many functions e.g. it may be instrumental as well as self-rewarding. Another function may be an attempt at cure.

Heather, referred to the clinic at age 9 as 'a severe case of stealing', had been 5 years old when her mother died of cancer, after having been nursed at home during a slowly developing illness. Within 2 weeks Heather had started school. Father kept the home going for Heather and her sister aged 8, but he was a quiet, rather withdrawn man, interested only in his work and in cycling, and he preferred the sporty Lyn. Heather had been close to her mother, and after her death she changed from a gay friendly child to a 'child you never notice'. This was how she was described at school where the sympathetic headmaster remarked 'I have never seen her smile'. Her pretty, unsmiling face stares out from a school group taken when she was 7.

It was from about this time that Healther started to steal; quite large sums of money, and always from father, who being absent-minded did not realise what was happening for some 18 months. With the money Heather bought dolls, dolls of every age, shape and size. She played with them at the house of a girl she knew slightly whose mother had once asked her in for a slice of cake and a glass of milk. In her play (later recreated in the clinic setting) she played the alternating roles of baby, child, teenager, and mother.

When Heather's father realised what had been happening to his money he was horrified, and the discovery of the cache of dolls did nothing to mollify him. He took Heather first to the headmaster, then to the Police and only on their advice accepted referral to the clinic.

## C. Response and Reaction

Although as we have seen any response is better than none, some responses are more favourable for the child than others. Sympathy and pity are felt for the child who shows a physical reaction such as the trembling or vomiting of the school refuser, for the child with the psychosomatic complaint, or for the child who is clearly timid and anxious. Children who sublimate successfully or who react by scrupulosity and overconformity or who are model pupils may be praised and set up as an example, yet these children are also disturbed.

At the other end of the scale are children who act antisocially, who lie and steal, who are cruel and aggressive; or those who are enuretic or encorpretic, all these arouse hostility or disgust, yet they too are disturbed.

The overt reaction to the behaviour does not always match the inner reaction. It has to do with social class and knowledge of facilities, but is in addition, personal and individual.

Clive's parents though shaken (and in private hostile to him) did not delay in taking him to the family doctor who promptly referred him to the clinic (p. 45), while the same offence committed by a working-class lad might well have landed him at court. The action of Heather's father was typical of the punitive and repressive attitude he exercised towards himself.

## D. Symptoms and Pathology

Many so-called symptoms are normal at certain stages of development and in children never referred to clinics, e.g. temper tantrums and masturbation (Kanner ([1])). Parental expectations, standards and personal problems may account for the referral of such children. I have had a child of 3 referred for 'enuresis', a child of 7 referred for stealing 'from her own money box' and another of the same age for stealing dog biscuits.

In Eisenberg's([2]) opinion 'The possibility exists that the difference between the child who appears at the clinic and the one who does not may lie less in the child than in the diagnostic perception of his parents and teachers.'

To make a further distinction it appears that parents and teachers often do not see the same child, either because children behave differently at home and at school or because parents and teachers pick out different aspects of behaviour to worry about.

The well-known (1966) Isle of Wight study by Rutter Graham([3]) of 10-year-old children in the population is very relevant in these matters. Parents and teachers were asked to rate their children on a check list of disorders of behaviour, and two child psychiatrists then examined a sample of the children to determine which of the children were maladjusted. The psychiatrists' ratings were inter-consistent, also all the children found to be disturbed by the psychiatrists had been found to have high symptom counts on the scale as rated by the teachers or the parents but not by both. The greatest difference occurred over the less objective symptoms such as withdrawal, solitariness, sadness. Thus it appears that parents and teachers do not see the same child but this does little to explain it. Other studies, e.g. Hewitt and Jenkins,([4]) seem to indicate that parents on the whole are concerned about the happiness and relationships of their children, and teachers about symptoms which have a loading of nuisance value which threaten discipline (disobedience, insolence, disruptiveness) or morals, (but parents may react protectively towards their children on these counts). Both parents and teachers are concerned about obstacles to learning. We have seen that middle-class and working-class parents will have different expectations from the clinic; now it appears that parents and teachers also have different hopes.

## E. Criteria for Diagnosis of Disturbance

'Symptom counts' have been mentioned, and clearly a child who presents with multiple symptoms, enuresis, pilfering, night terrors, temper tantrums, for example is likely to be disturbed, whereas a child with a robust personality, who presents with enuresis alone especially if there is a history of late acquisition of control in the family is unlikely to need referral. On the other hand one crippling symptom such as panic in crowded places such as the school assembly hall indicates a need for help; or even if the symptom is trivial and the parent is very concerned referral may be indicated on behalf of the parent.

The other pointer is the question of global disturbance, i.e. the general state of the child; an unhappy child, a child obviously carrying a burden or a child who 'acts out' wildly without any pleasure in his misdeeds, all are crying for help. A sudden change in behaviour without an obvious precipitating cause may be another sign.

## F. The Concept of Maladjustment

When a child is sufficiently disturbed as to require special educational treatment, it is necessary that he be 'deemed maladjusted' and recommended for special schooling.

The twin concept of education and treatment was developed as follows:

In 1946 the Ministry of Education described the children simply as being in need of 'special education' but in 1955 the Committee on Maladjusted Children[5] (a committee of educationalists) in the Underwood report, attempted to define maladjustment in more detail. They pointed out that it is not synonymous with aggression or troublesome conduct and delinquency although these might well be aspects of it. Rather 'insecurity and anxiety are closely linked with maladjustment' and such children are 'Insecure and unhappy in that they fail in their personal relationships.'

In 1946 the Ministry of Education took the step of fixing maladjustment as a medical concept since it recommended that child psychiatrists should refer such children to the school medical officers for ascertainment.

Warren[6] writes of the Underwood report, 'It has been criticised because its terms of reference confined it to so-called maladjusted children within the education system ... it missed the wider and deeper issues arising from emotional and mental ill-health among children and adolescents of all ages, the province of the Ministry of Health.'

Certainly the twin concept of education and treatment has not always been easy to implement for although the recommendation is made by the child psychiatrist, the decision regarding need and placement in a particular school is made by the education department, who often rely as much on the report of the headteacher as on the psychiatric assessment.

Gordon was a 12-year-old adopted boy from a middle-class family. He suffered from phobic problems (especially about eating food prepared by his adoptive mother) and also had bizarre ideas about his bodily functions. At home he often felt desperate, and this led to aggressive or even dangerous behaviour. At the secondary modern school he was very quiet and withdrawn, making no friends, but in no way a disciplinary problem. The recommendation for maladjusted school stressed the urgency. However the boy was put near the bottom of the waiting list on account of the report from the head-teacher which ended 'I have enquired from all the staff who teach him whether this boy requires a maladjusted school, and the unanimous answer has come "Certainly not" '. Since this seemed a strange conclusion regarding a boy with such severe problems, we discussed with the Head the idea which he and his staff had regarding maladjustment. It appeared that this was firmly equated with 'difficult behaviour', 'on the verge of delinquency', 'aggressiveness', 'antisocial behaviour' and they added 'and we have many like that in the school who really need a special school'. This was not an isolated view, for on enquiry we found that it was held by a cross section of head-teachers, though heads of primary schools were more likely to add 'children who are worried and anxious'. It seems to reflect the preoccupation of heads of secondary schools in particular with violence and problems of discipline.

In addition educationalists decide the policy regarding the maladjusted schools run by their department, and appoint staff. If a child psychiatrist attends he is likely to have little say in matters of these kind or about admissions and discharges. Independently-run schools which cater in whole or in part for maladjusted children who may be sponsored by local education committees are of course in a different position.

On-going discussion is centred around the whole concept of maladjustment; should there be two categories, social and emotional, should the whole concept be scrapped, should the recommendation be simply for a particular kind of schooling? This controversy also surrounds the question of doing away with other specific categories of disability, such as spasticity (cerebral palsy), autism, dyslexia.

## Bibliography and Further Reading

Items marked * are particularly important sources.

1. Kanner, L. (1960) Do behavioural symptoms always indicate psychopathology? *J. Child Psychol. Psychiat.* **1**, 1, 17–25.
*2. Eisenberg, L. (1961) The strategic deployment of the child psychiatrist in preventive psychiatry, *J. Child Psychol. Psychiat.* **2**, 4, 229–241.
3. Rutter, M. and Graham, P. (1966) (Isle of Wight Study) Psychiatric disorders in 10- 11-year-old children, *Proc. Roy. Soc. Med.* **59**, 382–387.
*4. Hewitt, L. E. and Jenkins, R. L. (1946) *Fundamental Patterns of Maladjustment: The Dynamics of their Origin,* Michigan Child Guidance Institute, Springfield, Illinois.
5. *The Report of the Committee on Maladjusted Children* (1955) (The Underwood Report), H.M.S.O., London.
*6. Warren, W. (1971) You can never plan the future by the past, *J. Child Psychol. Psychiat.* **11**, 4, 241–257.

## CHAPTER 7

# Classification and Diagnosis

The many attempts to formulate and classify childhood psychiatric problems indicate the complexity of the task.

In 1967 an 'International Seminar on the Diagnosis of Psychiatric Disease in Childhood', met under the sponsorship of the World Health Organisation (Rutter[1]). This was a multinational and multidisciplinary exercise by clinicians in the field.

The age range considered was 0 to 12 and a tri-axial classification (clinical psychiatric syndromes, intellectual functioning, etiology) was started, to be refined and elaborated at future seminars (the question of etiology was barely touched on).

From the suggested groupings I have dealt with some topics briefly, and have selected others for more detailed treatment. I have included relevant neurological conditions which were not included by the Seminar.

*Clinical Psychiatric Syndromes**

| | |
|---|---|
| Normal Variation | Neurotic Disorders |
| Adaptation Reaction | Childhood Psychoses |
| Specific Development Disorder | Psychosomatic Conditions |
| Conduct Disorders | Mixed |
| Personality Disorders | Subnormality |

## A. Normal Variation

Defined as 'Personality differences and emotional reactions within the range of normality', are common in childhood, and especially in the first 3

*M. Rutter has now outlined a five point classification as follows, Psychiatric Abnormality, Intellectual Level, Biological Disturbances, Developmental Disorders, Psycho/Social Problems (to be discussed at the next International Seminar in 1975).

years of life. An example is separation anxiety, and this and other transient problems may arouse parental concern, as may conditions included in the next two following categories.

## B. Adaptation Reaction
### (previously labelled reactive disorder)

This applies where although the symptoms are in excess of a normal variation there is no significant distortion of the child's development. An element of emotional stress is usually involved which may be acute or cumulative, the important point being how the child perceives the stress. Although the symptoms may be quite florid the condition is benign, provided the normal maturational and curative processes are facilitated.

Glen was an intelligent 9-year-old boy referred becausing of soiling, because he had the idea that a man was following him and thought he heard voices calling his name. He was preoccupied with death and asked his mother to make sure he had a gravestone. There had been three deaths in Glen's family; a baby sister found dead in her cot when he was 2½, his older sister Jane died of leukaemia a year before the referral and paternal grandfather, who had always lived with them, 3 months later. The family then moved to a new house and it was there that Glen's symptoms developed.

Jane, 3 years older than Glen, had been a second mother to him, taking him to school when he was small and fighting his battles for him. She had died after a short illness. Glen was sent to school on the day of her funeral (the parents confessed 'It was hard enough for us without him being there') and he had never been to her grave. The parents could see that they had bypassed Glen's mourning and to some extent their own; they were sensitive to his needs. Mother had given birth to a baby boy shortly after Jane's death, and her ability to help Glen with his complex emotional reactions was put to the test when she heard him saying to the 10-months-old baby 'Mother made Jane die'. However she was able to do this and in addition a supportive network of relatives assisted the family.

Glen's own robust personality was also an asset. He had plenty of friends, enjoyed outdoor pursuits especially football. He had made his own attempts to deal with his problem. He realised that he felt better at school or playing with his friends, and worse at home especially if inactive, or shut in a room with mother and the new baby Alan. So he went off with his friends, and when at home kept busy or sought out his father for a walk or a kick up at football. At night he would shut his eyes tightly so he would not know the exact moment when the bright light in his bedroom was put out leaving him with the shadows from the dim landing light.

He made full use of the opportunities in the clinic to play, and ventilate his feelings about Jane's death, his guilt for his imagined part in it and for his wish that someone else had died, perhaps his mother or Alan. He spoke of his part-welcome of the voice which was said to be Jane's voice, but which he was now hearing less often.

Both Glen and his whole family worked hard at his cure, and in 3 months all his symptoms had gone, and had not recurred at a 2-year followup.

## C. Specific Developmental Disorders

This category is reserved for biological delays and distortions of maturation. The conditions are more common in boys than in girls. They may be mild or severe, and secondary emotional disturbance is usually due to problems of handling. Some of these conditions e.g. stammering, and 'dyslexia' are discussed in a later section.

*Neurotic disorders, disorders of conduct and personality*

Most suggested classifications of childhood psychiatric disturbance, e.g. Rutter([2]), have distinguished between those affecting personality (sometimes called neurotic disturbance) and those affecting conduct.

The 1967 Seminar also separated clear-cut neurotic disorders, but made a further distinction between personality disorders and conduct disorders. (The two latter categories carry a poor long-term prognosis as shown by Pritchard and Graham's([3]) 1965 study of patients who had attended the Maudsley Hospital both as children and as adults. See also Rutter and Graham,([4]) Wolff,([5]) and Hunt([6]).

## D. Neurotic Disorders*

These are among the commonest problems referred to child guidance clinics. The child may present with frank anxiety, fears particularly at night or actual nightmares, worry in the face of change or mildly stressful circumstances, or clinging, regressive behaviour and enuresis. Children vary

*See Escalona,([7]) Isaacs,([8]) and Freud, A.([9])

tremendously in their ability to tolerate anxiety-provoking situations, depending on constitution, the way they have perceived previous experience, degree of maturity and so on. Very young children do not have the experience to know when anxiety is relevant to a situation, and parents and significant others in the child's life have a part to play in treading a middle path between over-caution and foolhardiness, and in monitoring anxiety for the child. If the parent is anxious, the child readily becomes anxious too, and a pattern is likely to be set up.

Neurotic symptoms may also be a defence against anxiety which is aroused not so much by real situations as from a conflict between the child's inner needs and impulses and the demands of the external world. We have already described how defence mechanisms are brought into play, but it is important to recall here that the child's armoury against anxiety is weak, and he is not adept at the use of defence mechanisms. Where they are in use, a secondary gain may be that some aspects of the child's development such as social adaptation and learning are allowed to proceed, but if defence mechanisms break down while the personality is still weak there is likely to be an end to constructive growth. Instead the child regresses and wallows in the mud of infantile struggles and rivalries.

A common defence is the projection of anxiety onto some object, person or animal, and the child experiences anxiety when faced with the phobic object.

Paul, aged 12, lived with his father, mother, and younger sister. They were an intellectual middle-class family, father a university lecturer, mother a teacher before marriage. There was a history of instability on mother's side of the family, and she had suffered from phobic symptoms as a child. Paul showed marked obsessional rituals at about 4½ before starting school, where he found it hard to settle. Now at a prestigious grammar school he is competitive and successful.

For the past 18 months he has shown fears of dog's excreta and of contamination, death and disease, handwashing and other complicated rituals have developed at home where all his symptoms are worse. He has a tense relationship with his mother and mutual irritability and rivalry with his sister. He has no close friend, but is able to take part in rugby, scouting, camping in connection with school, and to go sailing with his father.

Another and more painless 'escape' is for the child to develop hysterical conversion symptoms, weakness or paralysis of a limb, pain related to the abdomen, to the limbs or some specific organ such as the ear, or hysterical aphonia. These may be grafted onto an existing physical condition.

Robert had suffered from asthma from the age of 2, and later from sinus trouble and swollen glands in his neck. He had always been overprotected by his mother who paid frequent visits to his school to ensure that the teachers were aware of his fragile state. He had two older sisters, the next to him 5 years older. He failed the selection examination at 11, but after an enquiry had been pressed through by the parents, he was placed in a grammar school. Robert did not find the academic work easy and in addition was unable to cope with the normal ragging first-year pupils had to meet. In a playful scuffle outside school two boys tugged on the woolly scarf which Robert wore round his neck. On arrival home he had lost his voice. In spite of intensive investigations, no organic cause was found for this.

### E. Conduct Disorders

Here there is a long-standing disturbance of behaviour, which is often, but not always, criminal (hence the deprecation by the Seminar of the use of the expression antisocial as synonymous with conduct disorders) but which in any case indicates a disregard for feelings; thus such behaviour as sadism and cruelty (to humans or animals).

The behaviour must also be abnormal in its socio-cultural setting. Associated with this behaviour and apparent from an early age is a difficulty in personal relationships. This state is thought to be a 'lack' rather than an illness arising not so much from what went wrong as from what never went right. We find as we would expect a family background of rejection, often by both parents, with a lack of mothering and great frustration of basic needs. An impoverishment of personality organisation results (week ego, poorly developed superego). The problems of conduct result from a lack of inbuilt control, either controls have never been learnt or they have not been sufficiently consolidated so that they give way under ordinary stresses and appetites inherent in living. There is an inability to control the frontier between thoughts, phantasies and action.

A characteristic of children with character disorders is that they apparently feel no guilt and that they tend to repeat the same behaviour. This had been thought to be a masochistic seeking of punishment but P. Scott considers that the maladaptive behaviour as a whole arises because the child was trapped in a situation where excessive punishment, individual discrimination and confinement (within the family) produce (as it has been shown to do in animals) maladaptive repetitive behaviour. There may also be a need for control and care (being looked after).

It has been suggested that conduct disorders may be associated with delayed or defective maturation of the central nervous system and in some cases this can be corroborated by electroencephalographic recordings.

## F. Personality disorders
(some prefer the term character disorder)

This too is a longstanding condition in which the patient continues to act out conflicts belonging to the stage of early childhood. Relationships are used to fill a dependent or aggressive need, so that deep mutually caring relationships are not formed. As they grow older these children may strive to make other children scapegoats and when they become parents may encourage their children in anti-social or anti-authority or promiscuous acts. Thus another cycle is perpetuated through the generations.

## G. Delinquency

It is thought appropriate to introduce the subject of criminal and anti-social behaviour at this point. (Seminal works by Aichhorn,[10] Burt[11].)

Delinquency is a symptom rather than a category of disturbance. It may denote family or cultural influences, conduct or personality disorder, or as we shall see it may be an aspect of neurosis. It has a multifactorial etiology and attempts have been made to distinguish subgroups as an aid to prognosis and treatment.

### Hewitt and Jenkins[20]*

*Maladaptive.* This group is close to conduct disorder characterised by early and severe parental rejection. The child has poor peer group relationships and poor personality organisation and is sullen, vengeful and suspicious.

*Adaptive.* In contrast these children show physical vigour, a positive and aggressive attitude to life and good peer group relationships. For a time they have known good maternal care which has allowed the development of social responsiveness, but there has been a lack of consistent discipline and of parental guidance, especially a lack of interest from the father who may have

*For more details of psychosocial aspects see Bowlby,[12] Little,[13] Miller,[14] O'Kelly,[15] Stott,[16] and Gibson.[17] For more details of congenital and organic factors see Stott[18] and Pond.[19]

been absent for long periods. The home is usually cramped and disorderly and the boy either stays out or is cast out, often living with his street companions.

*Subcultural.* This has sometimes been called the 'sour grapes' group being found especially in high density areas especially where there is high youthful unemployment, and where delinquent behaviour is the pattern. In addition some of the children may be acting out a parent's personality disorder.

*Untrained group.* These children come from families which are grossly disorganised; the lack or inconsistency of discipline arises from the parents being undisciplined, but they are loving and accepting of the child.

*Delinquency as an Aspect of Neuroses.* P. Scott[21] discusses adaptive delinquency and points out that delinquent behaviour may be a means of adjusting to a stressful situation. Many emotionally disturbed children may show pilfering as one of their symptoms. A more complex mechanism is what he calls reparative behaviour (or conditioned avoidance reaction). Here the child attempts to find a new behaviour pattern or role in order to adjust to some stress in his life situation. This may be a socially acceptable life style or it may be stealing, fetishism or homosexuality.

### Grant and Grant[22]

*Classification by integration levels.* Influenced by the propositions of Piaget[23] and Erikson,[24] these workers have evolved a social maturity scale based on the development hurdles which the individual has surmounted, from which predictions are made in great detail regarding treatment requirements (regime, kind of therapist, etc.). Seven stages are described: level 1, the small totally dependent baby; level 2, totally egocentric, with other individuals seen purely as suppliers or withholders of wants; at level 3, others are seen as available for manipulation but not as having needs of their own; at level 4, there is a primitive conscience with crude white/black, good/bad differentiation; at level 5, there begins to be a true awareness of the needs of others and a sympathy with them; and at level 6 and 7, with a finer differentiation of conscience neurotic conflicts are the rule.

Grant and Grant conceive the development of a 'life style' based on the stage of development which the individual has reached, which serves as a defence against stressful or threatening situations.

*Relevance for Treatment.* Levels 2–5 are most often found among the delinquent population, and it is expected the psychotherapy will only prove relevant at the higher levels of integration. Indeed Grant and Grant consider that it is damaging to treat individuals in groups lower than 3 or 4 by counselling methods as they respond better to a strict authoritarian regime.

These predictions have been confirmed by studies carried out on institution-alised juvenile delinquents in California by Grant and Adams.([25]) At intermediate levels (or in the 'adaptive' group where there has been deviant identification) institutionalisation may not be necessary. It may be sufficient to keep the individual out of the delinquent subculture (where he is accepted) and re-establish him in a non-delinquent environment. On an out-patient basis this may be done by persistent thwarting of his delinquent activities and by honest emotional interchange and support from a probation officer who will help to enlarge his loyalty group to include socialised persons. At levels 5, 6 and 7 (mainly neurotic reactions) group or individual psychotherapy is rele-vant; Scott considers that for the 'reparative' groups special methods to reduce anxiety by the release of phantasy, and the introduction of more acceptable roles are suitable.

The greatest problem is the maladaptive group (level of integration group 2, conduct disorders).

Scott([21]) claims that such a child asks himself these questions, 'Am I an individual in my own right who can exist independently at all? Can I dare to make a relationship or to trust anyone at all? Does all loving involve attacking or being attacked? Being as I am how can I avoid hating myself? I know what I want to be like, but how can I start towards anything so distant and unattainable?' For these children there is a lack of basic trust in human relations and constancy. The best that can be hoped for them is that the placement does not make things worse for them. They need a structured situation in which it is clear what is expected of them, where they know that they will not fail (again), and have to move on somewhere else. It is clear that a group orientated permissive establishment may be too threatening for him.

*Application of learning theory to the treatment of delinquents*

Eysenck([26]) has suggested that delinquents tend to have a characteristic body structure. They are solidly built, heavy and muscular, and often show psychomotor clumsiness. (See also Glueck & Glueck([27]). He describes two groups, one usually extroverted who condition poorly, which includes a greater number of delinquents ; and a smaller group of more neurotic individuals who are responsive to conditioning, and who may have reacted to stress by learning a delinquent and deviant way of life.

The second group should respond to retraining programmes using con-ditioning techniques, but the first group would require prior medication with an extroverting drug such as amphetamine, after which they should respond to a socialising programme, including operant conditioning. These suppositions were not confirmed by Robin in his study of approved-school boys.

Eysenck suggests that aversion techniques (conditioned avoidance) may be utilised where alcoholism, other forms of addiction or sexual inversion or fixation complicate the problem.

### Martin

This case is presented as a follow-up to the above considerations of diagnosis and treatment.

Martin, aged 12, was referred to the clinic by the Headmaster of his secondary modern school for aggressive behaviour and truanting. The head was preparing to exclude him. He had already been 'excluded' from cubs, junior cadets, gym class and Sunday school and during the time we knew him was in fact excluded from two secondary schools.

He was the second child in the family with one sister older and two younger, and virtually the only male in the family since his father was in prison at the time of his birth and the parents separated soon after. Father would 'turn up' from time to time and on the last occasion gave Martin a dud cheque to go on a school trip. Mother was hostile to Martin and openly sided with the girls against him, but egged him on in his feuds with authority. She knew that he smoked and hung around to get lifts from lorry drivers to go 'all over the country', but was glad of the peace when he was out of the way. It had 'all gone on so long with Martin, from the time he started truanting from school and stealing from Woolworth's when he was 7'. Mother herself kept busy; among other things she worked as a home help for blind ladies.

In the clinic Martin was friendly and chatty. He bragged about the plaster 'pot' on his arm from a recent accident when he fell from a lorry, and how he 'made hell' for the nurses in the hospital, and threw his jelly at them. The same kind of behaviour occurred at school. His attitude was totally egocentric: he should be free to do as he pleases, anyone who gets in his way is 'for it'. As for his father: 'That pig of a gaolbird, all he ever did was give me a cheque that bounced.'

Martin was given to doing kind acts 'When I feel like it' such as helping old ladies across the road, but at other times he would laugh at cripples and kick out at dogs and cats.

## H. Addiction

Often an aspect of delinquency addiction is a symptom rather than a category of disturbance. It may also be an aspect of a conduct or personality disorder. It may even be thought of as a normal variation. Addiction in the young is especially thought of in connection with drugs, although addiction to alcohol and tobacco is also showing an upward tendency of late in both this country and the USA and should give great, if not equal, cause for concern.

'Soft' drug-taking often starts among adolescents (and the age is getting younger) in a similar way to the use of alcohol and tobacco as a social activity especially at parties, and for many it stays at that. For some, especially those who feel inadequate or underprivileged or who wish to rebel against society in general or the standards of their parents in particular, it may become all of life. Both the effect of the drug (euphoriant in the case of marijuana and amphetamine, and mind expanding in the case of lysergic acid diethylamide) and the shared drug culture appeal to inadequate, immature and unstable young people who may feel a closeness and belonging they have not previously experienced. Even the 'pet names' used for the drugs and for the methods of administration give the feeling of belonging to a kind of secret society. Addiction to these 'soft' drugs is more psychological than physiological. Dangers arise from the effect of some of them which may cause the taker to become intoxicated, so that he is unsafe at the wheel of a car or may do some rash act, and more specifically from the risk of a psychotic state (with amphetamine and LSD). There may be progression to 'hard' drugs which do induce a true physiological dependence. This usually occurs in vulnerable persons owing to exposure to the total drug culture, including the 'pushers'.

All types of addiction may lead to secondary delinquency, usually stealing to obtain money for the drug, but particularly with 'hard' drugs as the craving is so great. (It was hoped that this would become unnecessary with the registration of addicts but it has been only partly successful.)

Possession as well as usage of these drugs is of course an offence in itself, and there has been a lobby in favour of the legalising of marijuana, since it is said to be non-addictive and produces a gentle noncombative euphoria. It is also claimed that if it could be sold over the counter progression to hard drugs would be reduced. However, it has been said that marijuana is smoked just because it is forbidden and because the establishment regards it as decadent and dangerous, and that if this were changed a more dangerous drug would take its place.

This brings us back to the motivation for drugtaking and the fact that as well as treatment for the addiction itself the patient requires help with the social or personality problems which have caused him to become addicted.

## Bibliography and Further Reading

Items marked * are particularly important sources. Unnumbered references provide alternative sources to the references quoted immediately above.

1.  Rutter, M. *et al.* (1969) A tri-axial classification of mental disorders in childhood: an international study, *J. Child Psychol. Psychiat.* **10**, 1, 41–61.
2.  Rutter, M. (1965) Classification and categorisation in child psychiatry, *J. Child Psychol. Psychiat.* **6**, 2, 71–83.
3.  Pritchard, M. and Graham, P. (1965) quoted by M. Rutter in Classification and categorisation in child psychiatry, *ibid.*
4.  Rutter, M. and Graham, P. (1966) (Isle of Wight Study) Psychiatric disorder in 10- and 11-year-old children, *Proc. Roy. Soc. Med.* **59**, 382–387.
5.  Wolff, S. (1967) Behavioural characteristics of primary-school children referred to a psychiatric department, *Br. J. Psychiat.* **113**, 8, 885–895.
6.  Hunt, J. McV. (1944) *Personality and the Behaviour Disorders,* Ronald Press, New York.
7.  Bergman, P. and Escalona, S. (1949) Unusual sensitivities in very young children, *Psychoanal. Study Child* **3–4**, 121–140.
8.  Isaacs, S. (1932) Some notes on the incidence of neurotic difficulties in young children, *Br. J. educ. Psychol.* **2**, 1, 71–91.
*9.  Freud, A. (1962) Assessment of childhood disturbances, *Psychoanal. Study Child,* **17**, 149–158.
*10.  Aichhorn, A. (1951) (1st edition), *Wayward Youth,* Imago (English edition) London.
11.  Burt, C. (1925) *The Young Delinquent,* London University Press, London.
12.  Bowlby, J. (1946) *Forty-four Juvenile Thieves,* Balliere, Tindall & Cox, London.
13.  Little, A. (1965) Parental deprivation, separation and crime, *Br. J. Crim.* **5**, 4, 419–30.
14.  Miller, D. (1964) *Growth to Freedom,* Tavistock Publications, London.
15.  O'Kelly, E. (1955) Some observations on relationships between delinquent girls and their parents, *Br. J. med. Psychol.* **28**, 59–66.
16.  Stott, D. H. (1962) Sociological and psychological explanations of delinquency, *Int. J. soc. Psychiat.* Congress Edition, **4**.
17.  Gibson, H. B. (1969) Early delinquency in relation to broken homes, *J. Child Psychol. Psychiat.* **10**, 3, 195–204.
18.  Stott, D. H. (1962) Evidence for a congenital factor in maladjustment and delinquency, *Am. J. Psychiat.* **118**, 9, 781–794.
19.  Pond, D. A. (1961) Psychiatric aspects of epileptic and brain-damaged children, *Br. med. J.* **2**, 1377–1382, 1454–1459.
20.  Hewitt, L. E. and Jenkins, R. L. (1946) *Fundamental Patterns of Maladjustment, The Dynamics of their Origin,* Springfield, Illinois.
21.  Scott, P. D. (1965) Delinquency, in *Modern Perspectives in Child Psychiatry,* (ed. Howells, J.) Oliver & Boyd, Edinburgh.

*22. Grant, J. D. and Grant, M. Q. (1959) A group dynamic approach to the treatment of non-conformists in the navy, *An. Am. Acad.* **322**, 125–135.

*23. Piaget, J. (1932) *The Moral Judgement of the Child*, Routledge & Kegan Paul, London.

24. Erikson, E. H. (1959) *Identity and the Life Cycle*, Psychological Issues, Monograph 1, International Universities Press, New York.

25. Grant, J. D. and Adams, S. (1962) *The PICO Project: The Sociology of Crime and Delinquency*, Wiley, New York.

26. Eysenck, H. J. (1964) *Crime and Personality*, Routledge & Kegan Paul, London.

27. Glueck, S. and Glueck, E. T. (1950) *Unravelling Juvenile Delinquency*, The Commonwealth Fund, New York.

## CHAPTER 8

# Persistent Refusal to Attend School

I have chosen to deal with this problem in some detail, because of its topical interest (especially in view of the raising of the school leaving age), because of its importance as underlined by the Seebohm Committee, and because of the misconceptions which still arise, bedevilling communications between the different agencies and persons working with the child and the parents.

Until the late 1930s children who failed to attend school in the absence of physical illness were classed as truants and dealt with as though they were naughty or delinquent. In 1932 a neurotic condition distinct from truancy was described by Broadwin,[1] and this relatively rare condition has engaged the interest and concern of those involved in the welfare and education of children ever since. Recently the wheel has turned full circle and one school of thought considers that it is disadvantageous to distinguish between school refusal and truancy, since the former is then regarded as an illness requiring understanding and treatment and the latter a misdemeanour requiring punitive methods, with scant regard for the situation in which the child finds himself.

However, following our studies of delinquency it does seem useful to distinguish between truancy as perhaps a social ill leading to a conduct disorder and school refusal as a neurotic state; for the same method of treatment will not be applicable to both. Recent studies have in fact been along the lines of further subdivision of the school refusal group with the aim of clarifying their needs (Hersov,[2] Berg[3]).

Profiles of truants and school refusers will point the differences.

## A. Truancy

John had several separations from his mother during infancy and his father was absent or working away from home for 2 years after John was 4. He has had five changes of school. His standard of work is poor — 'he couldn't care less'. His IQ (85) is in the dull range and his attainments 2 years retarded. At school he is cheeky and independent, well regarded by his peers. He has one older brother working away, an older sister at an ESN school, and three younger siblings. Sometimes he stays at home to look after them (this form of absence is sometimes called 'school withdrawal') as mother is working part-time. He gives the impression that his parents don't rate school highly, they do not 'show up on open days' or enquire about his progress, they don't know when he is off school. John's general health is good. When he stays away it isn't because he is ill but because he has something better to do, or he got up late, or one of his mates is off; anyway he doesn't think much of school, 'what's the point, me Mum and Dad got on well enough without much schooling'. He has a better time roaming the town with his mates 'nicking' bottles off doorsteps, or 'some stuff from Woolworth's, a bit of a laugh. What's the fuss about anyway?'

## B. School Refusal

Clive, aged 12. He had only one separation from mother, but she is neurotic and overprotective towards Clive; father opts out. He has one sister aged 18, working from home but engaged. Clive only changed from infants to junior, from junior to secondary modern (mother had hoped for a selective school). Clive always found it hard to get to school. On the first day at infants he thought 'What will mother do without me?' He often cried and had odd days off, and longer periods after a holiday or a minor illness. Since transfer he has been more absent than present. He gets ready to go, then feels sick, dizzy or has a headache, but is better by mid-morning. He used sometimes to set off for school and return at the right time hiding during the day in his grandfather's allotment shed or even at the end of his own garden. He didn't try that again once his parents found out. They have struggled physically and emotionally to get him to attend but he fights them, runs off or becomes so distressed that they feel it is brutal to proceed. Clive is quite happy staying at home; he doesn't see his friends from school now, 'I help mother. Mother takes me out'. When at school he doesn't take part in activities and mother often writes a note asking for him to be excused PE, swimming or football. His standard of work is slightly ahead of his age group except in Maths. (His IQ is 112).

Clive would like to be able to attend school and comments that he usually feels 'alright when I get there and my parents have left'. He worries about not going, but even more about attempts to get him to go. His attitude towards the clinic is a mixture of the same timidity and aggressiveness which he shows towards mother. On his first appointment with me mother kept Clive close to her, holding onto his sleeve as she steered him towards my room, then half hanging on, half pushing him off, she urged him 'Talk to the lady', and aside to me 'He won't tell you anything unless I'm there.' Clive rounded angrily on her saying, 'I won't talk to either of you', entered my room and banged the door.

## 1. Diagnosis of school refusal

It is important to be able to distinguish school refusal from other conditions where failure to attend school is also a part, such as truancy, neurosis, psychosis.

Berg[3] has suggested the following criteria: severe difficulty in attending school often amounting to prolonged absence, plus severe emotional upset (possibly with somatic symptoms) staying at home on schooldays with the parents' knowledge at some stage, and the absence of antisocial disorders.

Other factors often, though not always, present are excessive dependency on mother, and above average (or at least average) intelligence. Certainly most of the children are conscientious workers and good achievers, but this probably reflects parental attitudes.

The emotional upset often takes the form of timidity and fearfulness outside the home and timidity with temper tantrums at home.

## 2. Categories of school refusal

### Acute and chronic

The acute cases start suddenly with at least a 3 year gap from previous school attendance difficulties, are usually in younger children and relatively often in girls. The chronic cases have a more insidious onset and appear in older children, usually boys. (Coolidge,[4] Berg,[3] Warren[5].)

Berg,[3] studying early adolescent children, has noted that the children in the chronic subgroup show a greater attachment to mother and less freedom of movement away from home.

*Neurotic (neurotic crisis) and characterological (way of life) phobia*

These two groups have been described by various writers (Kahn and Nursten,[6,7] Coolidge[4]) under their various names and broadly coincide with the acute and chronic groups.

In the neurotic type the personality remains intact and the child functions well in other areas (rather like the phobic condition of Paul). The characterological process seems the culmination of a relentless development during which the child has given up the attempt to form relationships or act independently although there may be occasional and petulant attempts to break free. These children are often adolescent and both Hersov[8] and Coolidge[9] have stressed that the condition can be particularly damaging at this time of life.

In most of these cases there is evidence that the child has a poorly organised personality, and has failed to develop ego strengths to enable him to deal with the demands of the outside world. Nor has he the standards (superego) to allow him to see the need for the (reasonable) structure which the school sets up. The whole school 'thing' with its routines and traditions are alien to him (and often to his parents also), and not only alien but also threatening and draining from him what little reality contact he has, especially in secondary school.

*School refusal as an aspect of underlying conditions*

School refusal may appear as one aspect of a neurotic or of a psychotic condition. Here it is necessary to concentrate on the underlying condition and these cases are not included here.

### 3. Misconceptions and red herrings

*The school's point of view*

Clive's headmaster summed up his bewilderment by saying, 'I can't understand it, he's one of my best boys.' By this he meant that the lad was intelligent, worked well and kept up to standard in spite of absences, and that when he was in school he settled down and seemed 'all right'. He desperately wanted to help Clive, to get him to attend school and be 'normal' but in his bewilderment he tended to assume that since school wasn't the problem it must be handling at home and told the parents they should 'deal with it'. This was greatly resented.

## The education welfare officer's point of view

He sees a different picture, having witnessed the parent's struggles to get the boy to school, the boy's evident distress and his own failure in the face of what seems at the time 'real illness', but he may also notice that Clive is manipulative and domineering with his parents, and that his mother, although so keen to get the boy to school, tends to raise difficulties just as he is about to depart. Also, particularly if the boy comes from an area where there is a 'subculture of truancy', he may fear the reaction of the other boys if Clive is seen to be 'getting away with it'. He tends to end up between the school and the parents, pleasing neither.

## The parents' point of view.

They (the mother especially) point to the boy's wish to be at school, his obvious distress and physical illness when he attempts to go, and the reasonableness of his worries; a shy boy, he is embarrassed at being seen naked; a gentle boy, he doesn't like rough games; a boy pushed him into the swimming pool, a prefect shouted at him, the maths teacher won't stop to explain, and so on and so on. And when and if these things are changed, the parents still feel that the wrong thing was changed or in the wrong way while the school feel exasperated that after all their trouble the boy still isn't in school.

## The point of view of the family doctor

It is not easy for the family Doctor to come down firmly with a diagnosis of school refusal in a child who suffers from frequent minor illnesses, or prolonged convalescence. The mother is usually at hand to detail the child's symptoms or relapse and the child may look pale, ill and trembly. For a long while the mother may conceal the fact that the symptoms clear up by mid-morning and that they never occur at weekends or during the holidays. Neither child nor mother may focus on any difficulties at school. It is only when the doctor feels that 'this time' the boy really should get back to school that the true nature of the condition is revealed.

Early diagnosis is important however, because a cooperative attack on school refusal in Bristol showed that when paediatricians and family doctors picked out children 'at risk' and involved the child guidance clinic team, so that preventive or early treatment was instituted, there was a significant fall in the number of cases (Kennedy[10]).

## 4. Predisposing and trigger factors

### School factors

Most of the children do focus on certain aspects of school (some of the common ones have been mentioned) and it is not disputed that children who are immature, unintegrated or mother-tied may have particular difficulties about situations in school which present them with the possibility of failure and which leave them exposed in some way (See Berg,[11] Moore[12] and Stott[13]). The name given originally to the condition, 'school phobia', accepted the child's assessment of the situation, i.e. that he was afraid of school. This view is still held by some workers, particularly the behaviourists and Eysenck and Rachman[14] have distinguished between cases where there is a true avoidance reaction and phobia for school which they consider to be quite common and the remainder which should be called 'separation anxiety in a school situation'. Most clinicians however would consider that in a sense the school 'problems' are red herrings, i.e. they obscure the true dynamics of the situation, though clearly if the child is experiencing real difficulties these should be corrected. But often when examined more clearly they are seen to have meanings not related to school.

### Home factors

These children find it particularly difficult to get to school if there is particular stress or illness in the family; if father is unemployed, mother ill or having an operation, or if there are marital tensions or quarrels. All these put an additional strain on the child and may tip the balance between him being able to get to school or not, since they threaten his slender security and increase his fears of what may happen at home while he is away.

## 5. Secondary effects on the child

The focusing of anxious attention on him and the conflict of opinion of which he is usually well aware cause the child to become more disturbed. His parents try to force him to go to school, yet try to change things in his environment to please him. They veer from a punitive attitude to a smothering, loving one, or show opposing attitudes. At school the behaviour of pupils and teachers may vary towards him according to whether they feel sympathetic towards him or not. Moreover the regime which he is supposed to follow may be changed in an arbitrary manner. He knows that his parents resent the school's attitude. The result is that he has a feeling of power without security, and some of his anger, dominance and manipulative behaviour may arise from this. The effect is often to withdraw sympathy from him. A rather sinister development is his withdrawal from outside contacts. For a time the child may go out and see his friends out of school hours, at weekends and during holidays, later only when it is dark, finally not at all, reaching the 'hermit stage' when he stays in his house or his room doing nothing and seeing nobody.

## 6. Causation and psychopathology

Here we are dealing with the neurotic type of school refusal. The point has emerged that the school problems do not represent the basic cause of the condition but that anxiety which belongs somewhere else is projected onto the school.

### Mother and Child

Most researchers and clinicians have considered that the nub of the problem lies here. Something has gone wrong in the early formative years so that mother and child have not been wholly freed from the symbiotic relationship. It has been said that the school refuser is 'not so much a schoolphobe as a motherphile'. Is the child's over-attachment to the mother [dependence], and inability to separate from her without anxiety due to deep affection for her? Certain remarks would suggest this. Clive: 'I just want to be at home with my mother'. Or Geoffrey, recently transferred to grammar school in the town: 'I just think of mother all the time when I'm at school. My junior school in the village was just across the road from our house, and I could peep and see mother moving about sometimes'. Yet a closer scrutiny might suggest another explanation. Clive: 'I wondered what mother would do without me', and Geoffrey: 'I worry that something might happen to my mother when I'm not there, I always have. In the village it wasn't so bad'. These remarks suggest a fear that some harm might befall mother and are reminiscent of the anxiety generated in young children by their hostile thoughts and their attempts to combat this by magic rituals and even the development of transient phobias. Transient because the need is transient, and most young children are able to work through their feelings of ambivalence towards their parents. It is the negative aspect of the ambivalence which the school refusers seem to have been unable to deal with (and the parent too). Davidson([15]) has stressed the primitive quality of the ambivalence which is seen in the school refuser, with love and hate existing side by side. Mothers who have problems in their relationships with their husbands, who have been or who are themselves phobic, may invest too much in their child, thus becoming overprotective or having a great need for their child's presence. For the child's part it would explain why if the mother becomes ill or if marital difficulties are overt the child feels unable to leave her. Johnson[16] has described this in detail and notes the particular relevance to adolescence. We can see that it is not only the change of school and general environment but also the beginning of the partly-welcomed strivings for independence which threaten both the child and the parent. When dependency and ambivalence have not been fully resolved, the child doubts his ability to fulfil a more grown-up role, feels guilty about wishing for even a small measure of autonomy, while the parents (especially mother) fear they are losing their child who will now be exposed to the dangers of the world outside the family. So both child and parent in their panicky state welcome a return to a more childish stage when everything was 'simple'. In this light we can see how the 'double-bind' behaviour of the mother arises and the effect it has on the child especially in early adolescence. His anger, petulance and stubbornness, and especially his refusal to attend school, give him the feeling that to some extent he is asserting himself and taking charge of his own life; but his behaviour which turns people against him rallies his mother to his side and he accepts this with clinging dependence.

This explanation also gives meaning to some of the specific school problems, exemplified by the cases of two children who had some distance to travel to their secondary schools, and who were both afraid of missing their transport. Mark refused school only on Mondays. On that day he was expected to go on a cross country run during the last periods of the afternoon. This took him some way from the school premises where the taxi to take him home would arrive sharp at 4 o'clock. Mark was not a robust boy and he feared that he would not be able to get back to the school in time from the farthest point of the run. He had tried turning back half way, but was ridiculed by the other children.

Barbara was also afraid she would not reach home. Each day she scanned the skies and listened anxiously to the weather forecasts, and at the least hint of rain, fog or snow she would feel unable to leave for school, as 'I might not be able to get back home'.

Bowlby[17] points to the importance of real stresses in the child's life, usually connected with family and home, in the genesis of the school refusal. He also divides the cases into four types, and so considers that they require different treatment approaches.

1. Mother, or more rarely father retains child at home to be a companion.
2. Child fears something terrible will happen to mother or father while he is at school so stays home.
3. He fears something terrible will happen to him while away, so remains.
4. Mother, rarely Father, fears something will happen to child so keeps him at home.

*The family, father's role* (See Bowlby([17]) and Skynner([26]))

We have noted that there has been a reaction against the focus on the pathogenicity of the mothers to the exclusion of fathers, and certainly Hersov([8]) (and Davidson,([15]) Nursten([18]) and others) have called school refusal a whole family problem. Herzov found excessive attachment to the mothers in only 50 per cent of his fifty cases. In his series there were three main family groupings.

Mother indulgent, overprotective and father passive, child dominant.

Mother demanding, severe and controlling, father passive, opting out, child timid.

Father dominant, mother insecure, child uncertain (a small number).

In many of the families the father is dismissed by both mother and child as irrelevant; though not physically absent he is absent as a power in the family. In the case of Clive, when the social worker visited the home in the evening with the expressed intention of seeing father, the latter withdrew into the kitchen leaving her with mother and Clive.

In cases where the father is the involved parent, academic pressures often figure prominently or the fathers are rather effeminate and take on a nurturing role, often having been school phobic themselves, and tending to identify with the child.

Norman, aged 9, on first referral was the youngest of three children and the only boy. Mother worked full time and was the dominant parent. Father who had had many changes of job was described by mother as 'an old woman'. He used to tremble as he described Norman's symptoms which were the same as he had suffered over getting to school when he was a child. Norman's symptoms had started when he moved from infants to junior school, now his worry was focused on 'the decimal point'. Father, frustrated himself academically, was very ambitious for Norman, and wanted him to get to grammar school, although he had been warned that the boy's intelligence was only borderline, and, since he was tense and a worrier, that he might do better at the top of the secondary modern. Father gave in to Norman and tried to organise an easy life for him since any stress 'might ruin his chances at the 11 plus'. Norman began to improve a little. Father was taking him to school, and felt that time attending the clinic might also affect his chances, so we did not see them again until Norman had been at the grammar school for two terms. Now he was refusing school completely, having been totally unable to settle into an environment more demanding both academically and socially. Father became emotionally upset, and there was marked hostility between Norman and Mother.

Davidson[15] has stressed the importance of treating the whole family and has pointed out that if one child in the family presents with school refusal and either is 'cured' or goes to a residential school, another child may develop the problem.

## Mother and daughter

Wilson[19] in particular refined the picture in regard to mother/daughter relationships, and found that there was often a three-generation bind of maternal grandmother, mother, daughter with both a need and a resentment of the need operating in all three, and with the grandmother often living in the home. Father is either absent or takes a passive role.

Shirley, aged 8, was refusing school. Father had left home 2 years previously and mother suffered from depression with some paranoid features. Two older brothers had left home. Mother attempts to get Shirley to school but on the way there one or other of them break down or feel ill and they have to return home. Maternal grandmother, who lived with them, used to tell mother she was cruel to Shirley when she tried to get her to school.

## 7. Treatment*

Treatment of children who refuse to attend school is a complex matter for a number of reasons.

Although the symptom (failure to attend school) is the same, the state of the child and the underlying dynamics differ. In addition the same symptom is shown in truancy. Various interested parties are hovering on the brink of the clinic, their hopes and expectations depending on their view point and motivation as outlined above. They only 'come together' in their wish to see the child back at school and thus behaving normally. A good deal of pressure is put on the clinic to achieve this. Yet the duty of the clinic team is to the child and family, and one of the first decisions which may have to be taken is

*See Davidson[15] and Waldfogel.[20]

whether to try to get the child back to school by whatever means or whether to put this question on one side for the time being and treat the underlying problems. In this case it is essential to explain to the interested parties what is being done and why.

Long-term treatment (psychotherapy) of the child (and/or family) would seem to be the treatment of choice in neurotic children, with return to school as part of the eventual aim. Those involved may find it difficult to accept and implement this because of the need to see the child in school, but if efforts to get the child to school (tried already so long and so hard) continue, partial success may seem to indicate that the problem is over, and in the event of failure the focus is still on how to get him there.

During psychotherapy, and with the focus off school, the child may suddenly say 'I think I'll go to school next week', or, casually, 'Ive been going to school since Monday'. This of course does not mean that treatment is at an end.

In acute neurotic cases there may be a case for immediate return to school, if it can be arranged with the cooperation of the headmaster that school is administered 'in small doses' and that the child is encouraged after even a short attendance or a visit to begin with and that this small success is not seen as a reason for stepping up expectations too rapidly. Alternatively flooding (p. 28) may be used. It is likely that there will be long-term failure and relapse unless co-incident and follow-up treatment and support is instituted for the family.

However it is children with personality (character) disorders who most benefit from a graduated return to school under a planned regime. These are children who (lacking ego strengths) are unable to face the reality of life in general and school in particular. They need to be able to start off all over again with small doses of school, and with authority figures with whom they can identify without fear. Skill and patience are needed on the part of the clinic team to interpret this need to the school and to support them during its implementation. Where there is a lack not so much of contact but of confidence in the clinic the school may become discouraged (especially with a boy who shows anger and manipulativeness as well as anxiety) by the setbacks which are bound to occur, and suddenly institute a more forceful and even punitive regime. A factor in this decision is also the fear (which we discussed in connection with the school welfare officer) of appearing ineffectual in relation to what 'this boy is getting away with'.

Where the condition has been long-standing a residential school may be needed to fulfil the same role. Here, with 'home' and school on the same campus, with a choice of adult figures with whom to work out identity problems, and opportunities to try out peer group relationships in a relatively sheltered environment, these children often do well (Warren([21])).

Where residential treatment is used, it is essential for therapy to be continued with the child and family during holidays and on follow-up after his return home if he is not to relapse (Weiss and Cain([22])).

Family treatment may well become the treatment of choice for these problems, and the student may choose to think this through by reading the section on family therapy at this point. Resistance to this approach must be expected on the part of a family who 'just want to get our son back to school', and since the treatment will reveal and expose the underlying faulty dynamics of the family, the family needs to have some strengths.

Follow-up studies have been carried out by Roderiguez,([23]) Coolidge,([24]) Warren([21]), Skynner([26]) and Berg([25]).

## 8. Postscript

### Raising of school leaving age

The impact of the change has fallen most on the first group of children compelled to remain at school until after their 16th birthday. Many who have during most of their secondary school years expected to leave at 15 have tended to deny the knowledge that they must remain, talking as though they were leaving or at least as though there was still some hope or some way of 'getting out of it'.

Those who have been disenchanted with their secondary school experiences, especially those in the lower streams, and those most in trouble for disciplinary offences, are loudest in protest. Not being able to hit out at the legislators who are really to blame, they act out in the school or community often in an extreme manner. Some of these arrive at child guidance clinics because the parents or the school are concerned at their attitude or behaviour or because the latter has led them into some trouble.

It is doubtful whether child guidance can do much to help these school-children who want to be adult workers — an 'assessment centre' may be able to 'hold' them.*

---

*By the 'Education Work Experience Act' of 1973 during the last year at a comprehensive school certain children may undertake certain types of employment if approved by their Local Education Authority.

*Children who are rejected by school*

If we think of the school refuser as rejecting school, the child who is excluded from school may be thought of as having been rejected by the school. Some of these will be the group described above, others are usually the children who act violently and who are disciplinary problems. Such a child may be a scapegoat or fall guy set up for his role by the other pupils, or he may be seeking some status for himself with his peers by cheeky exploits or mildly delinquent exploits. He is always the one who gets caught. 'John Jones again', says everyone. Some episode, the culmination of many, is the last straw and the headmaster excludes the boy or threatens to do so. He may be aware that home problems are disturbing the boy, but this only confirms his opinion that 'this is not a school problem'. Child guidance may be requested.

Here again it is difficult to know in what way it is possible to help. Some education authorities have made special efforts to deal with this problem. In one town children of all ages who the heads feel it necessary to suspend or exclude from school are offered attendance at the child guidance and remedial centre for a period of 3 weeks, during which time the staff of the centre work with the children, and are also in touch with the school and with the family. Some are referred for further assessment. A full assessment of this project is not ready, but it appears that a good proportion of the children are able to return to school. An alternative is setting up special assessment centres to help schools with their problem pupils and that has been done with success in some areas. It is thought that there should be at least two teachers, and a welfare assistant, and that there should be adequate space indoors and out for recreational as well as classroom activities.

A few children attend full-time, but most are part-time and may attend the ordinary school also; eventual aim is return to school, but not necessarily the same school.

### Bibliography and Further Reading

Items marked * are particularly important sources. Unnumbered references provide alternative sources to the references quoted immediately above.

1.　　Broadwin, I. T. (1932) A contribution to the study of truancy, *Am. J. Orthopsychiat*, **2**, 253–259.
　　　Patridge, J. (1930) Truancy, *J. ment. Sci.* **85**, 45–81.
　　　Eisenberg, L. (1958) School Phobia: A study in the communication of anxiety, *Am. J. Psychiat.* **114**, 712–718.

*2.   Hersov, L. A. (1960A) Refusal to go to school, *J. Child Psychol. Psychiat.* **1**, 2, 137–145.

3.    Berg, I. *et al.* (1969) School phobia: its classification and relationship to dependency, *J. Child Psychol. Psychiat.* **10**, 2, 123–142.

*4.   Coolidge, J. C. *et al.* (1957) School phobia – neurotic crisis or way of life? *Am. J. Orthopsychiat*, **27**, 296–306.

5.    Warren, W. (1948) Acute neurotic breakdown in children with refusal to go to school, *Archs. Dis. Childh.* **18**, 266–272.

*6.   Kahn, J. H. and Nursten, J. P. (1962) School refusal: A comprehensive view of school phobia and other failures of school attendance, *Am. J. Orthopsychiat.* **32**, 3, 707–718.

*7.   Kahn, J. H. and Nursten, J. P. (1968) *Unwillingly to School,* 2nd edn:., Pergamon Press, Oxford.

*8.   Hersov, L. A. (1960) Persistent non-attendance at school, *J. Child Psychol. Psychiat.* **1**, 2, 130–136.

*9.   Coolidge, J. C. *et al.* (1960) School phobia in adolescence: a manifestation of severe character disturbance, *Am. J. Orthopsychiat.* **30**, 3, 599–607.

10.   Kennedy, W. A. (1965) School phobia: a rapid treatment of fifty cases. *J. Ab. Psychol.* **70**, 4, 285–289.

11.   Berg, I. (1966) A note on observations of young children with their mothers in a child psychiatric clinic, *J. Child Psychol. Psychiat.* **7**, 1, 69–73.

12.   Moore, T. (1966) Difficulties of the ordinary child in adjusting to primary school, *J. Child Psychol. Psychiat.* **7**, 1, 17–38.

13.   Stott, D. (1966) *The Social Adjustment of Children,* University of London Press, London.

      Kahn, J. H. (1958) School refusal: some clinical and cultural aspects, *Med. Offr.* **100**, 137–139.

*14.  Eysenck, H. J. and Rachman, S. (1965) The application of learning theory to child psychiatry, in *Modern Perspectives in Child Psychiatry* (ed. Howells, J.) Oliver & Boyd, Edinburgh.

15.   Davidson, S. (1961) School phobia as a manifestation of family disturbance, *J. Child Psychol. Psychiat.* **1**, 4, 270–287.

*16.  Johnson, A. M. *et al.* (1941) School phobia, *Am. J. Orthopsychiat.* **11**, 702–712.

17.   Bowlby, J. (1973) *Attachment and Loss,* Vol. 2. *Separation: Anxiety and Anger,* Hogarth Press, London.

18.   Nursten, J. P. (1958) The background of children with school phobia, *Med. Offr.* **100**, 340–342.

19.   Wilson, M. C. (1955) Grandmother, mother and daughter in cases of school phobia, *Smith College Studies in Social Work,* **25**, 26.

20.   Waldfogel, S. *et al.* (1957) The development, meaning and management of school phobia, *Am. J. Orthopsychiat.* **27**, 4, 754–780.

21.   Warren, W. (1965) A study of adolescent psychiatric in-patients and the outcome six or more years later, *J. Child Psychol. Psychiat.* **6**, 1, 1–17.

22.   Weiss, M. and Cain, B. (1964) The residential treatment of children and adolescents with school phobia, *Am. J. Orthopsychiat.* **34**, 1, 103–112.

23.   Roderiguez, A. M. *et al.* (1949) The outcome of school phobia: a follow-up survey of 41 cases, *Am. J. Psychiat.* **116**, 540–544.

24.   Coolidge, J. C. *et al.* (1964) A ten-year follow up study of 66 school-phobic children, *Am. J. Orthopsychiat.* **34**, 3, 675–684.

25.   Berg, I. (1970) A follow-up study of school phobic adolescents admitted to an in-patient unit, *J. Child Psychol. Psychiat.* **11**, 37–47.

26.   Skynner, A.C.R. (1974) School phobia, a reappraisal, *Br. J. Med. Psychol.* **47**, 1–16.

## CHAPTER 9

# Psychoses in Childhood

## A. Early Infantile Autism

The first authoritative description was by Kanner[1] and I have used his name, although others have been suggested according to the experience and orientation of the writer; childhood psychosis, schizophrenic syndrome in childhood, aphasia with behaviour problems, etc. Great interest has been focused on the condition; in the early days after Kanner's description, children were 'discovered' in mental hospitals to be suffering from autism and some of these made dramatic improvements. The children themselves are usually 'bonny', with an alert look or a mysterious 'something' about them, and often with a special ability; all this suggests that if only the key could be found the child would develop its promise. Many children have been put forward by parents, educators, doctors and others as suffering from autism: in some the diagnosis has been in doubt, in others hopes of improvement have not been met.

### 1. Diagnosis

The incidence of the condition is in doubt, because of difficulty in establishing criteria for diagnosis. Wing[2] has differentiated between a 'nuclear group' (classical Kanner's syndrome) 2·1 per 10,000 and a non-nuclear group (not showing the complete classical picture) 2·4 per 10,000. This gives a total of 4·5 per 10,000, but some child psychiatrists would exclude some of the cases in the second group.

In 1961 a working party of clinicians, led by M. Creak,[3] spelled out the nine diagnostic points commonly found in autistic children. (The comments in brackets are mine.)

1. A sustained impairment of emotional relationships with people, including aloofness, empty clinging, using other people or parts of them impersonally. (This is the 'autistic' aloneness of Kanner, 'using people as things'. It tends to be most marked with strangers and in novel situations, especially outside home.)
2. Unusual behaviour towards his own body with scrutiny, exploration or self-directed aggression.
3. Pathological preoccupation with certain objects or parts of objects without regard to their accepted function (only part of a toy may be played with, such as the turning and turning of the wheel of an upended wheelbarrow. There is often a fascination with mechanical toys, especially screwing toys, and also jigsaw puzzles, and with particular objects, bits of material or string, which are manipulated endlessly. It is probably not appropriate to use the word 'play' for these activities.)
4. Resistance to change in the environment and a striving to maintain sameness: Kanner considered 'to produce a state of perpetual monotony'. (It is often selective, the child fixing on certain aspects of his life such as clothing, refusing to wear new clothes, or feeding, refusing everything except milk or crisps or apples, or routes taken in the car, the position of furniture or books in a room. The child becomes extremely upset if there is a change in this particular thing but not in others.)
5. Abnormal perceptual experience, the child showing visual and/or auditory avoidance, insensibility to pain and temperature, for example. (But they seem to feel cold easily, and they like to investigate by smelling, touching and other primitive means.)
6. Acute, excessive and seemingly illogical anxiety, which may be related to change or temporary interruptions of the symbiotic attachment to persons or things. (Everyday happenings may be invested with fear, such as the bathwater running out, or the telephone; but real danger does not provoke fear, and the children are often very daring, showing great ability to balance and climb.)
7. Speech. This may be arrested, lost or never acquired, and there are anomalies including repetition of words, phrases and questions, confusion of personal pronouns. (The answer to a question may be concrete. 'What would you do if you cut yourself?' 'Bleed'. The child may wonder about the whole business of communication, one intelligent 7-year-old quoted by Wing asked 'What do people talk for?')

8. Distortion in motility patterns, overactivity, immobility, posturing, rocking, spinning and ritualistic mannerisms. (The children appear to love movement, especially when it can be repeated, either by themselves such as on playground swings, slides or seesaws or by others, bouncing on a knee or swinging in the air, and in these situations the children appear animated, responsive and 'normal' but as soon as the activity ceases this fades.)

9. A background of serious retardation in which islets of normal, near normal or exceptional intellect or skill may appear. (The skill is often mathematical, musical or manipulative. Kenneth, aged 5½, at his first meeting with the psychologist asked him 'What is a parabola?'. The children often have excellent memories.)

## 2. Interpretation

Few child psychiatrists today would quarrel with this presentation of the clinical picture but the interpretations would vary. The main areas of divergence would be:

### Causation

Argument centres round the case for a psychological and an organic etiology. Kanner certainly considered that the 'aloneness' from which the rest of the abnormal behaviour stemmed was psychological and environmental, but Goldfarb[4] concluded that 50 per cent of his cases had an organic basis, and more recently O'Gorman[5] and J. K. Wing[2] have stressed the organic aspects, viewing autism as primarily a communication disorder. These workers see much of the behaviour of the autistic child as an attempt to find some order in the chaotic world which surrounds him, or as an attempt to preserve himself from interference from outside. They also point out that a similar condition to autism is seen in some cases of deteriorating brain disease where fatty substances accumulate in the brain. So far no organic pathology of the central nervous system has been found in children with autism when they have died of intercurrent disease.

Creak[6] has considered that the bizarre features of the condition suggest 'that this is a mental illness', but does not rule out organic factors.

### Intellectual functioning and learning

How intelligent are these children? Kanner thought that they had good intellectual potential but that their withdrawn state prevented them from utilising it: others consider that it is the disorder of speech and communication which does this. A comparison made by Wing([7]) of autistic, aphasic, partially sighted and control group children suggests that there are points of comparison between the abnormal children, and that techniques for teaching the other handicapped children could be modified for use with autistics. Nevertheless quite a large proportion (variously estimated from 30–50 per cent) are severely subnormal. Performance on intelligence tests is patchy, the relevance of formal intelligence testing has been doubted and special efforts have been made to find better ways of testing them, but there has been a correlation between tested intelligence and prognosis. In addition problems of attention and concentration and lack of motivation increase the learning problems.

## Onset

The original description was of an onset during the first 2 years of life. Many writers have considered that a period of normal development may precede the appearance of symptoms. However it appears that in most cases the child has been from the very early days puzzling, different, unresponsive, showing a failure to smile, or indicate readiness to be picked up, or to be 'cuddly', and later difficulties over feeding, toilet training and sleeping add up to a lack of intimacy and rapport.

## Subgroups

Mention has been made of the nuclear and non-nuclear group of Wing. Kolvin([8]) has distinguished an early 'classical' group of varying severity and a variable course and a 'late onset' group with a fairly rapid downhill course which he has named 'disintegrative psychosis'.

## 3. Family background and personality of parents

The parents of children diagnosed as autistic tend to come from social classes 1 and 2, and to include many professional, scientific and artistic individuals. A selection factor could operate here, especially in Kanner's early series. His original conclusions were that the parents (mothers especially) tended to be cold and intellectual, and he thought that handling might be a factor in the condition. On the whole this has not been confirmed. Creak([9]) found a cross section of personality types in the parents in her series; also that the attitudes of parents towards their autistic child were either that they enhanced the strangeness and also the special abilities of the child by making a way of life for the whole family around the child, and often identifying with him to some degree, or they tended to reject him. See also Klebanoff,([10]) Bettleheim,([11],[12]) Laig and Esterson.([13])

## 4. Prognosis

The prognosis is unfavourable if the tested IQ is below 50, if the child is not speaking by the age of 5, and if there is a high symptom count. Escalona has pointed out that these factors correlate highly with communication failure and teaching problems. Kolvin([8]) considers that late onset psychoses carry a poor prognosis.

## 5. Treatment and results

Whatever the causation, it must be accepted that autistic children suffer from severe and multiple handicaps.

### Keeping the child at home

If the parents are willing and able to cope, this provides the child with a predictable environment, and is likely to ameliorate at least some of his symptoms. Yet many families will not be able to deal with the punishing behaviour these children mete out. Wing([14]) has described this excellently and has also indicated the sort of adverse development which parents must expect, the reactions they may encounter, for example having the child who is having an anxiety tantrum called 'spoilt' because he looks so normal, advice about dealing with behaviour and finally the hope of improvement over the years.

Many families need relief from the total care of their child; a stable non-involved 'mother's help' may share the load more suitably than the more intellectual nanny, or attendance at a special day centre or school but in these schools, previously training centres, the staff need to be alerted to the needs of the autistic child.

### Treatment in special centres

*(i) Type of Centre.* Should the centre cater solely for autistic children, or should there be a mix with other handicapped children or with maladjusted children? Should the regime be mainly educational or mainly geared to social and psychological therapy? If the problem is thought to be based on communication and learning problems (probably with an organic basis) the setting

is likely to be educational, if on the other hand it is thought to be psychological, the emphasis will be on close personal contact probably in a nutrient and play situation. If the unit is small and special teaching techniques are used it is likely that the intake will be limited to like children, (see Bartak and Rutter[15]) but if it is part of a larger remedial or maladjusted set-up then it will probably be beneficial for the autistic children to mix for part of the day with children suffering from other forms of maladjustment and with normal children receiving remedial help. In this setting it is also possible to do away with the unfruitful dichotomy between education and psychotherapy, and for specialised teachers and therapists to work together to help the same children, so that improvement in contact and learning go hand in hand.

The odd speech of the speaking autistic child and his abnormal behaviour may be modified by a variety of measures including behaviour therapy. The child is promptly rewarded for appropriate speech and behaviour (imitative or spontaneous) and in some centres he is also punished for unacceptable speech and behaviour. (See Frith and Hermelin[16] and Geller.[17]).

*(ii) Day or Residential.* Residential treatment may be required if the condition is severe, if the child is severely subnormal or if the parents are unable to cope without detriment to the child and to family life as a whole. Units have been set up in connection with psychiatric hospitals, others in an educational setting. According to the severity of the condition and the special features of the handicap, the child may fit into a number of residential settings, schools for the educationally subnormal, or for mixed handicaps, maladjusted schools, schools for children with speech defects or aphasia and a number of others. A difficult child may be accepted at a Steiner school and may fit in there very well.

There is probably a tendency to move away from the concept of residential treatment for these children.

*Results*

When the child lives and learns in an environment which suits him, whether this is home or away there is often a slow spontaneous improvement with age, particularly in the sphere of relationships. M. Creak[6] found in her follow-up of 100 cases that 20 per cent improved sufficiently to attend ordinary schools at least for a time, and later to work, 20 per cent were able to live at home and attend a centre or sheltered workshop, a further 10 per cent showed some improvement. About 50 per cent did not improve. More varied treatment methods, and more facilities may show better results in the future.

## B. Variants, or Allied Conditions

### *Symbiotic psychosis*

Opinion differs as to whether this is a clear-cut condition. There is acute distress and anxiety at separation from mother sometimes from birth, at others arising between the ages of 2 and 5, often triggered off by the admission of mother or child to hospital. The children have always been a little 'odd' and close to mother. Temper tantrums usually develop, plus withdrawal and sometimes loss of speech and social regression. These cases are difficult to treat. Others seem to be reversible either with special help or where the family is supportive.

### *'Odd' children*

Another doubtful category.

The children never develop a true psychotic condition, but they stand out from other children mainly because they are social misfits within their peer group. Usually intelligent, they have some special bent or interest which they cultivate (and may be encouraged to cultivate by their parents) and which cuts them off from other children.

Bob had an interest in dinosaurs and this formed his sole topic of conversation. Aided and abetted by his father he had amassed a collection of pictures, models and literature.

The milder cases are labelled 'big head' the more severe 'screw loose'. In large classes the situation deteriorates, but the child may do quite well in a small remedial or maladjusted day group after which he is able to return to the ordinary school.

Valerie, aged 7, went through a stage of thinking she was a dog (or sometimes a cat). Her mother used to feed her dog or cat food, ('She'll only eat the kind advertised on TV') and gave her milk in a saucer on the floor. She objected, however, when Valerie wanted to be taken out for walks on a lead ('I only do it in the garden') or when she wanted to lift her leg against a tree (she appeared to think she was a male dog). She did, in fact, eschew femininity and insisted on wearing trousers. At school she would not play with the other children, called her headmaster 'Mr Squirrel' and often hid under his desk.

## C. Schizophrenia

This occurs occasionally in late childhood, and rather more commonly in adolescence. The symptoms are similar to adult schizophrenia with withdrawal ideas of reference and suspiciousness, unpredictable and impulsive behaviour. Hallucinations and bizarre ideas may develop. Suicide or attempted suicide may be the first sign of illness. Diagnosis is difficult. (See Stroh[18] and Bender[19].) Many adolescent breakdowns tend to be stormy and to have an 'odd' component. Also a depressive component may mask the underlying schizophrenic process.

## D. Depression

The frequency of true depression in early and middle childhood is a question about which child psychiatrists find it hard to agree. Some claim that it is rare, and that only in late childhood and adolescence does depression begin to appear. Others point to feeding disorders, withdrawal, prolonged 'mourning-type' reactions and learning blocks as an expression of depression.

Cytryn and McKnew[20] have described three types of depression occurring in children aged 6 to 12, masked depression, acute depressive reaction and chronic depressive reaction. Masked depression (hyperactivity, aggressive behaviour, psychosomatic illness, hypochondriasis and delinquency) appears in children whose histories reveal exaggerated stubbornness, and negativism (called by the authors 'passive-aggressive personality structure') and during their illness they displayed marked anger. Family members showed disorganisation and in some cases psychopathy.

Acute depressive reactions usually occur following a traumatic event in children with normal adjustment, involving loss of or change in relationship to an important figure. There is persistent sad affect, social withdrawal, hopelessness, retardation, sleep and eating disturbances. Chronic depressive reactions appear in children with a marginal and precarious adjustment who may have had depressive episodes previously, probably resulting from separations dating from early infancy; the clinical features are similar to the acute type but the child is excessively clinging and dependent. There is usually a history of depressive illness in the family and there may be a seesaw of depression between mother and child.

Frommer[21] studied 210 children under 5 referred to a child psychiatric department. 122 of these children showed signs of depression. There was a high incidence of precipitating factors, and a large number had depressed mothers. They were anxious, had sleep problems, reduced appetite and a significant number complained of abdominal pain.

In adolescence depression may be distinguished from normal 'moodiness' by its persistent character, by being worse in the morning and by being associated with feelings of guilt and sometimes thoughts of suicide.

Although depression in childhood is self-limiting and recovery is usual, it must be thought of as a serious condition on account of the danger to life from the anorexia and the risk of suicide especially in adolescence (Anthony and Scott[22], Despert.[23]

Antidepressant drugs are of limited use in childhood depressions but may be of value in adolescence.

## Bibliography and Further Reading

Items marked * are particularly important sources. Unnumbered references provide alternative sources to the references quoted immediately above.

1. Kanner, L. (1943) Autistic disturbances of affective contact, *Nerv. Child.* 2, 217–250.
2. Wing, J. K. (ed.) (1967) *Early Childhood Autism: Clinical Educational and Social Aspects,* Pergamon Press, Oxford.
*3. Creak, E. M. *et al.* 1961) Progress report of a working part – The schizophrenic syndrome in childhood, *Br. med. J.* 8, 89–90.
4. Goldfarb, W. (1961) *Childhood Schizophrenia,* Harvard University Press for the Commonwealth Fund, Cambridge.
5. O'Gorman, G. (1967) *The Nature of Childhood Autism,* Butterworths, London.
6. Creak, E. M. (1963) Childhood psychosis, *Br. J. Psychiat.* 109, 84–89.
7. Wing, L. (1969) The handicaps of autistic children: a comparative study, *J. Child Psychol. Psychiat.* 10, 1, 1–40.
8. Kolvin, I. *et al.* (1971) The phenomenology of childhood psychoses, *Br. J. Psychiat.* 118, 4, 385–395.
*9. Creak, E. M. and Ini, S. (1960) Families of psychotic children, *J. Child Psychol. Psychiat,* 1, 2, 156–175.
10. Klebanoff, L. B. (1959) Parental attitudes of mothers of schizophrenic, brain-injured and normal children, *Am. J. Orthopsychiat.* 29, 3, 445–454.
Menolascino, F. (1965) Autistic reactions in early childhood, *J. Child Psychol. Psychiat.* 6, 3/4, 203–218.
11. Bettelheim, B. (1950) *Love is not Enough – The Treatment of Emotionally Disturbed Children,* Free Press of Glencoe, Illinois.
12. Bettelheim, B. (1967) *The Empty Fortress – Infantile Autism and the Birth of the Self,* Macmillan, London.

13. Laing, R. and Esterson, A. (1964) *Sanity, Madness and the Family*, Tavistock Publications, London.
    Bateson, G. (1960) Minimal requirements for a theory of schizophrenia, *Archs. gen. Psychiat.* **2**, 477–491.
    Ackerman, N. (1961) The schizophrenic patient and his family relationships in *Mental Patients in Transition* (ed. Greenblatt, D. *et al.*), Charles C. Thomas, Springfield, Illinois.

*14. Wing, L. (1964) *Autistic Children: A Guide for Parents*, Constable, London.

15. Bartak, L. and Rutter, M. (1973) Special educational treatment of autistic children: a comparative study, *J. Child Psychol. Psychiat.* **14**, 3, 161–179.

16. Frith, P. and Hermelin, B. (1969) A developmental and behavioural approach to the treatment of pre-school autism, *J. Autistic Child*, **14**, 376–397.

17. Geller, J. (1972) The development of behaviour therapy with autistic children: a review, *J. chron. Dis.* **25/1**, 21–31.

18. Stroh, G. (1960) On the diagnosis of childhood psychosis, *J. Child Psychol. Psychiat.* **1**, 3, 238–243.

19. Bender, L. (1953) Childhood schizophrenia, *Psychiat. Q.* **27**, 663–681.

20. Cytryn, L. and McKnew, D. (1972) Proposed classification of childhood depression, *Am. J. Psychiat.* **129**, 149–155.

21. Frommer, E. A. (1968) Depressive illness in childhood, Chapter 10 in *Recent Development in Affective Disorders* (ed. Coppen, A.), Headley Brothers, Ashford, Kent.

*22. Anthony, E. J. and Scott, P. (1960) Manic-depressive psychosis in childhood, *J. Child Psychol Psychiat.* **1**, 1, 53–72.

23. Despert, J. L. (1952) Suicide and depression in children, *Nerv. Child*, **9**, 378–389.
    Scott, W. C. M. (1948) A psychoanalytic concept of the origin of depression, *Br. med. J.* **1**, 538–540.

## CHAPTER 10

# Constitutional and Organic Conditions which effect the functioning of the Child

This includes conditions with a neurological basis, and problems which are at least in part developmental.

## A. Mental Subnormality

In the past this has been seen as a separate speciality, but the present tendency is to link it to child psychiatry and paediatrics. The relevance to general medicine, neurology and genetics to subnormality is also established. Mental sub-normality has probably been the Cinderella of the medical sciences; it was considered an unrewarding speciality mainly because so little was known about it and it was assumed that little could be done. The position has changed and it is hoped that this section will reflect the change, although it is only possible to depict certain aspects out of a very wide field.

### 1. Changes in classification and legislation

Prior to April 1971 subnormal children were subdivided into educationally subnormal (IQ 50–70) and severely subnormal (IQ below 50), the former the responsibility of the education department as requiring special education, and the latter the province of the Ministry of Health requiring training. Since that date all subnormal children become the responsibility of the Department of Education and parents are entitled to claim education for them although there is a clause in the act excepting children unable to respond to an educational stimulus. This means that the named distinction between school and centre will be done away with, but it does not mean that training will cease to be required, it will continue as before alongside such education that the children can use for those IQ levels from 20–50.

Some special provision is needed for children with IQ below 20, for children who are severely subnormal and physically handicapped, and for disturbed subnormal children.

Special care units may continue to meet the needs of many of these children. Residential care will continue to be needed for some but it is considered that if the community services are fully developed, including parent support and the provision of hostel accommodation during the week, this would be greatly reduced, with the possibility of developing a more 'child orientated' regime in the hospitals.

## 2. Causation

### Genetic aspects

It is important to know something about the genetics of mental defect since parents to be may seek or need counselling because they know of an abnormality in their family, or because they already have an affected child.

Most inherited mental defect with an organic pathology is passed down according to Mendel's laws. In recessive transmission inheritance is indirect and parents are healthy carriers. If both parents are carriers then one in four of the offspring will suffer: phenylketonuria, the lipidoses, Schilder's disease and gargoylism (except for one type handed down by mothers to boys only) are examples.

In dominant transmission inheritance is direct, affected parents hand down the condition to the child, and 50 per cent of the children are likely to be affected. Tuberous sclerosis is an example, but most cases of this disease arise not from inheritance but from a new mutation, so parents who have had one child suffering from the disease may be encouraged to risk another pregnancy if they are both healthy.

### Mutations

These are changes in the patterns of genes, and unfavourable mutations are responsible for some cases of mental defect as we have seen in the case of tuberous sclerosis. Most mutations are said to be 'random' with no cause known, but may arise from radiation.

### Other forms of inheritance

Inheritance under Mendel's laws follow a pattern. In others errors occur sporadically as happens in the case of mongolism, and other conditions due to chromosome disorders. It is unusual for more than one mongol to be born into a family, but the risk is greater for mothers at the end of reproductive life (the 40–50 age group) and may then be as high as 1 in 40 live births, for a proportion abort spontaneously. Any disturbance in the chromosome pattern, except where it affects the sex chromosomes, is likely to effect the development of the brain.

*Other causes*

Interference with the developing foetus during pregnancy is most damaging in the early stages when growth is very rapid, either by infections (German measles, syphilis, viruses and toxoplasmosis from domestic pets) or radiation which may act directly on the chromosomes or initiate mutations. Nutritional defects during pregnancy in poorer mothers may cause the babies to be of small size, or these may show definite brain damage, and they are specially vulnerable to damage if they become jaundiced.

Damage at birth (continuum of reproductive casualty) may be from injury, haemorrhage, anoxia, and may cause cerebral palsy with mental defect.

The first 6 months while the brain is still developing is a danger period for all kinds of damage. Infections of the coverings of the brain (meningitis) or the matter (encephalitis) may result from bacilli or viruses. Tuberculous encephalitis and virus encephalitis (sleeping sickness) used to be fairly common, and the latter particularly caused deterioration of behaviour. The measles virus may cause catastrophic damage to the brain or a much slower mental deterioration. Injuries to the developing brain, however caused, may cause mental defect.

No cause is found for many cases of mental defect, but this does not imply that no cause will be found in the future. It is important to correct the frequent statement that most mentally subnormal children, especially of mild degree, are anatomically and physically normal. This was not borne out, for example, by the Isle of Wight study which provided evidence that many mildly mentally retarded children have handicaps additional to the mental defect.

*3. Pathology*

In some conditions the nerve cells of the brain (neurones) are gradually taken over by an abnormal substance (lipidosis and gargoylism are examples) the cause being a fault or lack of a particular enzyme. The children are normal at birth but the course is fairly rapidly downhill ending usually in very severe subnormality. Or there may be wasting of the white matter of the brain (e.g. Schilder's disease) due to a chemical error, with a similar downhill course and often visual and auditory deficiencies.

In tuberous sclerosis (epiloia) space-occupying abnormalities of the brain are present at birth, and the child often has epileptic fits.

The scarring left by encephalitis limits the possibility of improvement, but the condition is not progressive.

In mongolism (Down's syndrome) the deviation from normal growth is thought to occur early in pregnancy, and the brain is abnormal at birth, being small, rounded and more simplified than usual, with a poorly developed auditory area.

In phenylketonuria there is damage to the white matter of the brain which may become irreversible and is due to interference with an enzyme-facilitated chemical process. The accumulation of phenylalanine derived from the mother's milk (or cow's milk) causes damage which is not progressive, but which can be prevented if the right nutrient is provided for the baby especially during the first 6 months of life when the brain is developing fast.

In cretinism there is no genetic predisposition or chemical abnormality but a lack of thyroid, which if untreated leads to poor physical and mental development especially in the early years of life.

Damage at birth or in a road or other accident may lead to general mental defect as well as to cerebral palsy and defects of hearing or sight are also common.

In microcephaly there is a very small brain, as seen in mongolism and also in prematurity and where there has been poor nutrition during pregnancy, it can also be due to radiation and other causes.

At the other extreme in hydrocephaly the head is of normal size and shape at birth but later enlarges and may be enormous, out of all proportion to the body and becomes rounded. The extra space within the cranium is taken up by water and the brain thinned out. Some of the children have quite good intelligence however, but may suffer from other abnormalities.

## 4. Treatment

### Prevention

*(a) Genetic counselling.* The kind of situations where advice may or should be sought and the kind of advice which might be given have been

outlined: the remaining question is who should give it. It seems that it is appropriate for any medical person dealing with a family at the time when the need for counselling is felt should be in a position to give it; whether family doctor, obstetrician, paediatrician, geneticist, etc.

*(b) Education.* Particularly of the public, but also of the professions and the authorities. Knowledge of the dangers of a woman contracting German measles during pregnancy, of rhesus incompatibility and of phenyketonuria are quite common today among members of the public, and more people are interested in such topics.

*(c) Antenatal and Postnatal Care.* Certain measures are now routine; the investigation of the blood group of the expectant mother, and after the first child preparations for exchange transfusion made in the case of rhesus negative women (with Rh-positive husbands); the Wasserman test to exclude syphilis which although rare today has increased slightly of late; good nutrition, elimination of excessive work, etc.

*(d) Screening.*
1. Prenatal screening for blood group anomalies.
2. Routine screening for phenylketonuria before discharge from maternity ward or in the home.
3. Babies who are small and fail to thrive should be screened for protein-bound iodine for thyroid deficiency.
4. Routine screening of infants having fits, or 'at risk' from familial diseases.

*(e) Immunonology.* Prevention of measles, encephalitis.

*Treatment*

Treatment which is curative can be employed in phenylketonuria by a special diet which is vital during the first year and usually has to be continued until the child is 6.

In cretinism replacement therapy with thyroid may have to be continued throughout life.

Examples of the ways in which improvement may be achieved, for instance in mongolism, by the administration of serotopin which decreases the floppiness and treatment of the epileptic component in certain conditions.

## 5. Behaviour problems in mentally handicapped children

Some problems arise from the underlying conditions as in encephalitis, some from the awareness of the child that he cannot compete with his more able peers and some due to the reaction of the parents and their inability to accept the child for what he is. This is probably more difficult for parents of the mentally than the physically handicapped though both sets of parents have a problem in accepting an offspring who falls short of their ideal child and all the guilt and other emotions which are brought into play. The fact that the mentally handicapped child may also have an additional (but often unrecognised) physical handicap adds to the difficulty (see Rutter and Graham([1])).

The problem is probably greatest in all these aspects when the child is lightly handicapped (IQ in the 50–65 range). The child is more aware, and the parents have more conflicts, especially over the vexed question of whether the child should go away from home (see Rutter and Graham([1])).

Problems increase as the child grows older, especially if his normal physical appearance contrasts sharply with his behaviour, and parents feel embarrassed in many social situations and are at the mercy of tactless (though sometimes well-meaning) remarks much as the parents of autistic children are. If the child has been unwanted or adopted the problem is greater, or if the parents have a particular internalised need to have a perfect child. This does not mean that the parents are bad; they could have been perfectly adequate parents for a different child or in a different situation. Like the parents of Jo Egg they are caught in the tragedy of the situation.

It is the reality of the situation in which many parents find themselves which has to be faced. At one time a romantic name 'The Peter Pan Society' was suggested for what is now The Society for Mentally Handicapped Children. The first title ignored the fact that these children do grow up, and that parents of even young children worry about what will happen to them during their adolescence and adulthood.

## B. Gifted Children

Now that we have examined the problems of mentally handicapped children and their parents it may seem ridiculous to suggest that children at the other end of the intelligence range may have problems, but this kind of excellence may also be a potential stress. The children may be frustrated in the classroom, where in addition their quickness of mind and unchildish ways of thinking and speaking make them seem 'superior' to other children and even to their teachers. Often less mature emotionally, they may need play opportunities suited more to their chronological than to their mental age, but these become less accessible to them as other children ostracise them and grown-ups treat them like little adults. A role may be found for them as 'second teacher' but this encourages them still more to 'put away childish things'.

Discussion is still continuing as to whether it is wise to segregate and educate such children in special classes or in special schools, especially perhaps when they have a special ability (e.g. music).

## C. Organic Conditions of the Nervous System which Effect Behaviour and Learning

A number of conditions have been dealt with in the section on mental defect. A few further notes follow here.

### 1. Brain damage

We have seen that the immature brain of the foetus is especially vulnerable to damage. Certain brains seem to be more vulnerable to damage and there are also periods of optimum danger. One of these is the perinatal period, i.e. the period just before, during and after the time of birth. Toxaemias of pregnancy, drugs, birth injury, rhesus incompatibility and prematurity (especially associated with the immoderate use of oxygen) are just a few examples.

### Continuum of reproductive casualty

By this term Pasamanick[3] described damage which depends on the severity of the insult to the brain and the vulnerability of the particular brain. It ranges from abortion or stillbirth, through cerebral palsy with mental defect and epilepsy to minor degree of damage.

### Minimal brain damage (clumsy child) (see Clements and Peters[4])

The child shows poor coordination, catches and kicks a ball with difficulty, cannot tie shoelaces or do up buttons, and may have learning problems. There may be crossed laterality, i.e. may use his right hand for writing but kick with his left foot, and his left eye may be dominant. This causes additional confusion. It is important to diagnose this condition (which may be confirmed by finding 'soft' neurological signs, by EEG examination and by psychological tests including the Frostig so that parents and teachers may understand the very real difficulties which the child has, and which without this understanding might lead onto behaviour problems. It is not often that any 'cure' can be found but the findings may suggest teaching techniques which will help the child.

### 2. Epilepsy

In this condition the child experiences a loss or alteration of consciousness. It is due to abnormal activity of certain groups of brain cells, and this can be demonstrated on the encephalograph (EEG). There may be momentary clouding of consciousness (*petit mal*), or a generalised fit (*grand mal*). Even the latter type, frightening though the fits appear, may not lead to any alteration in the behaviour of the child, but if the fits are very severe or prolonged, or if they occur very frequently, it is likely that signs of brain damage will appear.

However, reactions of the parents in the way of overprotection or rejection and of others dealing with the child (at school) may lead to behaviour problems.

Focal epilepsy occurs when the abnormal activity is localised, and then local spasms or altered sensation result usually without loss of consciousness, but may spread to a generalised fit.

Epilepsy may be caused by some lesion of the brain or it may be idiopathic, i.e. the cause is unknown.

It appears that epileptic fits may occur when there is already brain damage, and also that damage may follow severe or repeated fits.

### Temporal lobe epilepsy

This is due to damage of the temporal lobe of the brain. The child may have a major fit or merely strange or frightening sensory or other experiences ('the aura'), and usually clouding but no loss of consciousness, but it may go on to a general fit. The children often show behaviour problems, particularly overactivity and sudden outbursts of rage, often when the child has been under mounting stress. It has been thought that these may be an attempt by the child to ward off attacks. Certainly they are very worrying and the child may sometimes be violent, and the reaction of concern mixed with hostility which they evoke will increase the stress on the child. Sometimes there are no dramatic signs, the child merely has a 'strange experience', then feels a little sleepy, and perhaps has a headache.

### Learning difficulties

These may be due to poor attention span and distractibility, or to mental retardation, or to a certain special attitude which is still sometimes shown to epileptic children even when their fits are well controlled. Epileptics with good intelligence are often conscientious and hard workers, and it has sometimes been considered that they drive themselves beyond a point which is safe for their neurological equipment. However an opposite point of view is that this, like the activity of the temporal lobe epileptic, is a 'fail safe' mechanism, and some studies have shown that when epileptics were put up a class and 'stretched' the number of fits declined.

### 3. Hyperkinetic syndrome (see Ounsted([5]))

There is overactivity, restlessness, poor attention and distractibility. Often there are behaviour problems such as aggression and disobedience. The symptoms usually appear before school age, but become an increasing problem as the child grows older, and the parents become distraught especially as the child sleeps poorly or wakes early. Learning difficulties are usual. Although this is an important syndrome, the term hyperkinesis is often used loosely and drug treatment which may be useful in the condition, but which may carry a certain danger, may be used inappropriately for a child who is merely restless, or just very active.

### 4. Syndrome of brain injury

This term was coined by Pond([6]) to describe the 'effect of unstable personality and subsequent environmental handling upon a child who as a result of brain injury is retarded in the general field of learning memory and intelligence'.

Bender([7]) has stated, 'even an organic brain does not create fundamentally new trends, but it merely underscores specific psychological problems'. This was confirmed by twin studies where one twin had a brain injury. The symptoms he showed were an exaggeration of the personality traits found in the uninjured twin.

In addition the home background, handling by parents, reaction of siblings, and attitude of teachers all have their effect.

Finally it is important to stress the tremendous recuperative powers which the brain has, with new areas taking over the function of damaged ones.

## Bibliography and Further Reading

Items marked * are particularly important sources. Unnumbered references provide alternative sources to the references quoted immediately above.

1.  Rutter, M. *et al.* (eds.) (1970) *Education, Health and Behaviour,* Longmans, London.
    Rutter, M. and Graham, P. (1966) (Isle of Wight Study), Psychiatric disorders in 10- and 11-year-old children, *Proc. Roy. Soc. Med.* 59, 382–387.
2.  Group for the Advancement of Psychiatry (1967) *Mild Mental Retardation,* New York.
3.  Pasamanick, B. (1961) Epidemiologic studies on the complications of pregnancy and the birth process in *Prevention of Mental Disorders in Children.* (ed. Caplan, G.) Tavistock Publications, London.
4.  Clements, S. D. and Peters, J. E. (1962) Minimal brain dysfunction in the school age child, *Archs. Gen. Psychiat.* 6, 3, 185–197.
5.  Ounsted, C. (1955) The hyperkinetic syndrome in epileptic children, *Lancet,* ii, 303–311.
6.  Pond, D. A. *et al.* (1963) Marriage and neurosis in a working class population, *Br. J. Psychiat.* 109, 592–598.
7;  Bender, L. (1961) Childhood schizophrenia and convulsive states, in *Advances in Biological Psychiatry* (ed. Wortis, J.), Plenum Press, New York.
*   Kirman, B. (1972) *The Mentally Handicapped Child,* Nelson, London.

## CHAPTER 11

# Developmental, Habit and Allied Disorders

## A. Enuresis and Encopresis

Wetting and soiling after the age at which control is normally established are common presenting symptoms in children referred to the clinic, but must be regarded as symptoms rather than clinical entities.

Although we speak of the normal or average age at which control is achieved, children vary widely; bowel control is normally achieved at least by about 3 years, and bladder control by 5 years, yet 10 per cent of children are still wetting the bed at 5 years, 5 per cent at 10 years and 1 or 2 per cent are still wet at night into their teens; particularly children who have never achieved control, the so-called 'continuous enuretics' (Miller,[1] Hallgren[2]).

Other children are 'trained' very early, even by 1 year, but are liable to relapse since voluntary control of bowel and bladder cannot be reliably achieved by the child until about 18 months. Up to that point it is the mother who is 'trained'. Unfortunately this is about the time that the child achieves greater autonomy and he may elect to rebel. This is one cause of 'discontinuous' enuresis (Apley and McKeith[3]).

As with other aspects of development there seem to be 'sensitive periods' for learning control of the bladder in particular, from 1½ to about 4 years. Subsequently 'training' may be more difficult to achieve (Cust,[4] Whiting[5] and Sears[6]).

*Subgroups*

*Continuous or primary enuresis or encopresis,* where control has never been achieved, is usually a developmental disorder (delayed neurological maturation) or a habit disorder (lack of or faulty training). There is a family history of similar trouble in about 70 per cent of the latter type.

*Discontinuous or secondary enuresis or encopresis* is usually a neurotic problem and the child shows other signs of disorder, or there has been a particular stress or series of stresses.

Anthony([7]) made a study of enuretics and encopretics and concluded that the continuous type was due to defective socialisation, while the discontinuous type was a neurotic disorder.

Anxiety is frequent among children with these problems; it may result from the reaction of parents and others to the condition or both the anxiety and the symptom may be part of a deeper disturbance.

*(i) Enuresis.* This is the commoner condition and is usually nocturnal (bedwetting) or may be diurnal, or both may occur. Daytime enuresis alone is uncommon and usually suggests an organic cause (abnormalities of bladder or urinary tract, infection, epilepsy or diabetes). Woodmansey([8]) suggests that discontinuous enuresis (or indeed encopresis) may occur initially 'by accident' or at a time when the child is under particular stress, and is then perpetuated by the reaction of the parents and by the child's conviction that he will never wake in a dry bed. Normally distention of the bladder initiates a reflex causing the child to awaken, and he becomes conditioned to that, but in the enuretic the reflex is never established (primary) or is lost through anxiety (secondary). Many of the neurotic children sleep deeply, but more continue to sleep because they fear to wake up once more in a wet bed.

Parents follow well-meaning advice or they initiate manoeuvres themselves, but restriction of fluids, 'lifting', restriction of activities such as family holidays, or camping trips with the scouts; all fail after a temporary success, as does bribery by giving stars for dry nights and similar methods. Parents try to ignore the symptom, but it is difficult to do this in face of the practical difficulties and the provocative and aggressive component which is often present.

Jane, aged 6, lived with her natural father, her stepmother (who had a son of about Jane's age) and two stepsiblings from the remarriage. Jane did not accept her stepmother. She was an intelligent child and showed a number of irritating symptoms including enuresis. Her father urged Jane to be 'nicer' to her stepmother. 'Make a special effort for Mother's Day', he said. Jane got up early and wrote 'Happy Mother's Day' in urine on the new wallpaper in her bedroom, then called her stepmother to see it.

At a deeper level, urine and faeces are the first things in his life over which a child has control, his first products, his first presents, or power, or magic or dangerous poison. Jane indicated in her play that she believed her faeces were poisonous and could cause harm.

*Treatment.* It is particularly important to exclude organic causes in diurnal enuresis and nocturnal encopresis, but once this has been done further examinations are to be deprecated.

Treatment with drugs is often useful in simple continuous enuresis, but should be supported by reassurance to the child and parent that the medicine will help the child to control his bladder function while asleep. Imiprimine or amitryptiline (antidepressant drugs) are useful but must be continued for at least 1 month after the child has become dry.

If drug treatment fails and particularly in older children who are well motivated, and in whom enuresis is the only symptom, conditioning treatment by the 'pad and buzzer' may be tried. The child sleeps in a bed in which metal sheets attached to a buzzer alarm are placed under his sheets and blankets. When he commences to urinate the buzzer sounds and the child wakes to find the bed only slightly wet. He is able to rise, urinate, reset the buzzer and he will reawaken should further urination occur. The repetition of the sequence conditioned stimulus urination buzzer enables the child to awaken before urination begins and confidence does the rest. Failures occur because training is stopped too soon (it should continue for 1 month after the child is dry) or because of lack of motivation in child or family, as either or both can 'sabotage' the treatment. Relapses do occur but a second course usually has speedy and lasting results. In cases where the family are inadequate a period in hospital for 'buzzer training' may be advisable.

*Discontinuous neurotic enuresis.* Woodmansey([9]) has stated 'it is not that something has to be done for the child, but that the child needs to be rescued from what is happening to him'. It is the concern of the parents about their child's elimination, and the measures they resort to to control it, which cause problems to continue.

The child is usually anxious and timid but there is often an undercurrent of aggression, as seen in the case of Jane, whose treatment was weekly psychotherapy, while the parents were seen by the social worker.

Treatment of parent(s) and child is usually along classical child guidance lines, looking at the motivation behind the symptom and focusing on the symptom, with the use of 'conditioning', is not usual.

*(ii) Encopresis.* Soiling is a less frequent but also a more serious symptom. Diurnal encopresis is the more common, and nocturnal more likely to indicate an organic basis (abnormality of the large bowel or anal fissure). Continuous soiling is usually due to lack of training in poor and inadequate families but the children function well otherwise. Discontinuous soiling is associated with emotional disturbance and disturbed family relationships.

Anthony([7]) found two types of maternal reaction in the neurotic cases; rigid obsessional mothers who overtrained with an anxious aggressive child and lax, indulgent mothers with a regressive reaction from the child.

Sometimes soiling alternates with constipation, since the child retains faeces and the soiling eventually consists of dribbling from overflow.

Stephen, nearly 6 when referred by the family doctor for soiling with constipation, was the middle of three boys. The two elder boys had become clean and dry exceptionally early. When Stephen was 2 and mother expecting the next child they were living in a strange town with father absent a good deal as he was on a course. Mother felt isolated and harassed. Both she and Stephen had an attack of diarrhoea which left Stephen with occasional loose stools which sometimes smeared his pants. Mother panicked, and punished Stephen every time this happened. Stephen responded by withholding his motions, even to the extent of sitting on a hard step; or he would go down the garden or into a corner of a shed to defaecate, or he would soil. Sometimes he would go as long as 3 weeks without a motion that mother could 'be certain of'. This was worse than the soiling, she became more and more worried, began to use laxatives and to beg the health visitor for enemas. Stephen liked apples and mother felt this was helping until he realised that she thought so and refused to eat another one. He hardly ever spoke to her and Mother felt that she and Stephen were 'at loggerheads'. She was an extremely conscientious but obsessional woman who desperately wanted to bring up her family well, and Stephen's bowel habits were a constant affront to her. What made matters worse was that he was quite normal and friendly at school where he was already 'doing well', and with other members of the family.

*Treatment.* Again investigation is only called for in a small number of cases. Most cases are of the neurotic type and here long-term treatment of child and family is indicated.

Occasionally massive retention of faeces indicates a short stay in hospital so that the bowel can be cleared out and the child and family given 'a fresh start', with, it is hoped, a non-punitive and hopeful attitude.

In continuous cases operant conditioning may be used. The child (who often will not even sit on the toilet but soils or defaecates in odd places) is encouraged at least to sit on the toilet. He is promptly rewarded for this. If he defaecates he is given a more imposing reward. It is easier to carry out this routine in hospital than in home, and a tolerant non-punitive attitude must be maintained.

## B. Feeding Problems

### 1. Refusal of food

Food refusal in young children is often the other end of the problem of soiling: the child is refusing to be rigidly controlled by what the mother considers he should eat. There is in addition a secondary gain from the attention focused on the child at mealtimes. All focusing on food should cease. There should be no special foods or coaxing, or eating up what has been left, or refusal to allow the child a preferred course until another has been eaten. Instead the normal food the family eats is offered at regular mealtimes for the child to eat or refuse. An alternative is to offer 'miniature meals', saying 'leave what you don't want'. Experimental work with young children who were offered buffet style meals over the period of a week showed that over the whole period the children chose a balanced diet. Similarly food fads and fussiness can safely be ignored.

These problems build up between mother and child, as we have seen in encopresis, until their relationship is centred round the food situation.

Anorexia nervosa is dealt with in the section on psychosomatic disorders.

### 2. Overeating

Overeating and the allied problem of obesity may have a physical cause such as endocrine, metabolic, (diabetes is an example) or may arise for emotional reasons. Deprived children may become thin, but they may also become fat, either because the child eats because he feels unloved, (and this may occur at particular times), or the rejecting parent may compensate by extra care about feeding (and dressing) the child well. A child may also eat through loving identification with a fat Mum or through rejection of a thin one (Bruch[10,11]). Some children eat to ward off depression.

Treatment varies according to the cause.

### 3. Pica

This is the eating of non-food substances, such as soil, wood, crayons, paint. It may cause lead poisoning and an important investigation in the United States began as an inquiry into why children ate the substances which produce lead poisoning.

Millican and Lourie([12]) found that, contrary to previous supposition, the condition was found in all social classes and usually indicated a disturbed mother-child relationship. It could develop as follows: adequate mothering is required to control the ingestion of food from about 5 months onwards and ingestion of unusual materials may relate to distortion of transitional phenomena due to inadequate mothering, and the children have other oral problems such as thumbsucking and feeding problems. They tend to be negativistic. Supportive and educational measures proved successful in a large number of the cases, psychotherapy of child and mother being required in only a few of the cases.

There was a suggestion that in many ways pica has the qualities of an addiction (distorted instinctual satisfaction) and a follow-up study will test this hypothesis (see also Cooper([13]) and Lourie([14])).

## C. Delay or Defects in the Acquisition of Speech or Reading

Speaking and reading must be regarded as communication skills, and problems arising may be due to organic or emotional causes or both.

### 1. Delay in development of speech*

For normal speech development a degree of maturation but also emotional rapport between the toddler and his mother (or surrogate mother) is required. Speech is one of the social skills which is rapidly lost when this contact fails, and mothers who are depressed or rejecting may be unable to provide it in the first place. A relatively rare condition, known as elective mutism, arises where the child chooses not to speak, or may cease to speak after, for example, the birth of a sibling, or may speak normally but only in certain situations (Reed([16])). Such a child may at quite a late age commence to speak spontaneously in a complicated sentence, such as Jane, aged 4, who unexpectedly said 'Won't someone please turn off the television?'. It is usually clear that the child understands what is being said. His non-speaking becomes a habit which it is hard for him to break especially as it has the advantage of focusing a great deal of attention on him.

Mental subnormality and organic brain disease are also causes of delay in speech development, and we have already described problems connected with speech in autism.

*See Morley.([15])

## 2. Abnormal speech

There may be immature speech, mispronunciations, aphasia or stammering. Immature speech as well as delay is often associated with difficulties in reading which appear later.

*Aphasia.* (Ingram([17])). In this condition, the child either does not understand the meaning of spoken words (receptive type) or he may understand but be unable to form speech (executive type). This is a severe handicap and the child may have to be taught by special methods, sometimes in a special school. The child may be thought to be deaf, or if he is intelligent he may learn to read and then the condition (or at least its severity) may be overlooked. It may be thought that he is acting or that he is 'naughty' when his understanding does not match up to his rote performance. Behaviour problems may result.

*Stammering.* (Andrews([18])). This condition is thought to be transiently normal in many children at about 2 years and later at about 5, in the form of slight speech hesitancies. As an established condition it is relatively common, being present in 4 per cent of children but more common in boys than in girls. It is thought to occur particularly in two categories of children; those in poor social circumstances, when it is often associated with low intelligence, birth trauma or low birth weight, and in children of good intelligence who have anxious driving parents (particularly mothers) when it may be associated with tics (habit spasms). In these cases the stammer often seems to develop from normal speech hesitancies when the parent (and later others) comment on it. 'The onset of stammer occurs not in the patient's mouth but in the parent's ear'.

## 3. Problems in learning to read and write

These too are communication skills, and children vary in their readiness to acquire them according to their intellectual capacity, central nervous system maturity and integration and emotional attitude.

*Dyslexia.* This popular word can indicate a number of things, but usually either a severe degree of retardation in reading (and usually also writing and spelling) of at least 2 years, and a condition sometimes called 'specific developmental dyslexia' thought to be due to a neurological condition. Not all neurologists and certainly not all educational psychologists accept this as a specific entity and if it does exist it is probably rare (Boder,([19]) Eisenberg([20])). The Advisory Council on Handicapped Children([21]) gave it as their opinion that it is preferable to use the term 'specific reading difficulties' to cover the small group of children whose reading (and perhaps spelling, writing and number) abilities are significantly below the standard which their abilities in other spheres would lead one to expect, and that the needs of these children are best considered as part of the wider problem of reading backwardness of all kinds.

(This would do away with the elitist category of specific dyslexia. Similar doubts have also been expressed about separating autistic children from the wider category of children with other difficulties of learning and communication and of separating cerebral palsy from the wider category of physically and mentally handicapped children.)

There is no doubt that bright children with problems in reading and allied skills do become frustrated, as do their teachers, and need help and understanding, and that particular techniques may have to be evolved to help them. It has been suggested that the term perceptual handicap could be applied to a number of them who have difficulties with reading or with number concepts, and that the refined techniques for diagnosis such as the Frostig test could be utilised more fully in pinpointing areas of difficulty and in the plan for remedial help (Bateman,[22] Alberman,[23] Tansley,[24] and Sheridan[25]).

Discussion also arises as to whether such help should be offered in the ordinary school, by withdrawal groups, on a sessional basis in a clinic or centre or for a full-time period at a remedial centre.

## 4. Educational pressure

Though not a disorder, this is a very common cause of unhappiness in children and often perpetuates the situation it aims at curing. Stimulation and encouragement are positive but pressure is usually negative and deadening. Both the educational system and the expectation of parents may produce it. Selection procedures for secondary education which have disappeared in their original form in all but a few areas probably made matters worse, but if one pressure is removed others may take its place. Parents wish to have successful children, children they can be 'proud of', and especially parents who had to miss the educational opportunities they see opening up before their children. Teachers may back this up or may take a more realistic view (see Jensen[26]).

Ruth, aged 13, was referred for difficulties in reading and spelling. She had had a number of changes of school. In her junior school she had difficulty in learning to read. She was thought to be deaf and when this was ruled out a period in a remedial centre was suggested. The parents turned this down since they felt she would be with children of a lower intellectual and social class. They sent her instead to a boarding school a long way from home where her work was said to improve but where she developed behaviour problems. With Ruth now at the secondary modern, soon to become comprehensive, father has 'persuaded' the headmaster to try her in a stream in which O levels as well as CSE are offered in order that 'Ruth can take at least Biology, English and History at O level'. He is incensed that they have advised she drops Maths, and quotes one exam at the boarding school when Ruth scored 90 per cent. Father had to leave school at 14. He is a successful self-made man, who has worked hard at night school and moved several times to further his career. He would have liked a son but is now determined that Ruth shall be successful since his elder daughter, once thought to be 'academically promising', is about to 'flop out' of art school.

Ruth wants to work outdoors with flowers and father is determined that she shall stay on at school after 16 and take a 'proper' course at horticultural college. Mother, a rather depressive woman, says that father has 'a bee in his bonnet' about education, but she herself finds Ruth very irritating and silly, 'fussing about little things', and much prefers the headstrong and flamboyant Julie.

Ruth's IQ was 93, just within the low average range. She had poor success with the performance tests which seemed to link with her difficulties in reading and writing. Her better verbal fluency was thought to reflect her family background. There was no evidence to point to a 'specific dyslexia or perceptual disorder'. Attainments in reading and spelling were very low, reading being 4 years and spelling 5 years retarded. Arithmetic was a little better and only 2 years retarded. Ruth felt very discouraged. 'Everyone gets onto me, especially about spelling, it's all getting worse. I don't want to go away. I hated that boarding school.' Then, 'The flowers won't know whether I can spell or not'. Ruth has found out that she can take a course at college without O levels, but father won't listen.

It certainly seemed as though father would not listen. The psychologist explained his findings to him in detail, but father just said that Ruth was a late developer just as he had been. (He had had no chance to develop, but Ruth had been given plenty of chances.) He felt that the school was rejecting Ruth (and him) and he had stopped going to see the teachers. Things looked black for Ruth. Still he did agree that the psychologist should contact the school and oversee Ruth's progress there, and after several of these visits and several visits from father to the psychologist, he suddenly announced that he had decided that Ruth should drop down a form, that she should take only

Art at O level, and that she should leave school at 16 and take the practical course at horticultural college.

*Late developer*

This term, like dyslexia, is often used as a face-saver. What is usually meant is that hidden potential is waiting to flower. When this does occur, as in the case of the late Winston Churchill, signs of good potential have usually been evident, but the child has not elected to use it.

Other children may progress slowly in all aspects of their development, and with maturity and a gain in confidence may be better able to harness what ability they have. When, however, the term is used in the case of an anxious child, such as Ruth, already becoming distressed and disturbed in attempts to meet parental standards it can only lead to worsening of the situation.

This is well described by Tolstoy in *Anna Karenina.*([2 7]) Seriozha, Anna's son, is failing in the academic work he does for his father and his tutor. He is pre-occupied with thoughts of his departed mother. 'In his father's opinion he did not try to learn what he was taught. As a matter of fact he could not learn it. He could not, because his soul was full of more urgent claims than those his father and the teacher made upon him ... He was 9-years-old, he was a child, but he knew his own soul and treasured it, and without the key of love he let no one into his heart. His teachers complained that he would not learn while his soul was thirsting for knowledge.'

## Bibliography and Further Reading

Items marked * are particularly important sources. Unnumbered references provide alternative sources to the references quoted immediately above.

1.  Miller, F. J. W. *et al.* (1960) *Growing up in Newcastle-upon-Tyne,* Oxford University Press, London.
2.  Hallgren, B. (1959) Enuresis in the child population, *Acta paediat.* Supplement No. 118, 66.
3.  Apley, J. and MacKeith, R. (1968) *The Child and his Symptoms,* Blackwell Scientific, Oxford.
4.  Cust, G. (1958) The epidemiology of nocturnal enuresis, *Lancet,* ii, 1167–1170. Shirley (1938) Encopresis in children, *J. Pediat.* 13, 267.
5.  Whiting, J. W. M. and Child, I. (1953) *Child Training and Personality,* Yale University Press, New Haven.
6.  Sears, R. R. *et al.* (1957) *Patterns of Child Rearing,* Row, Peterson & Co., Evanstown.
*   Pinkerton, P. (1958) Encopresis, *Archs. dis. Child* 33, 371.

*7. Anthony, E. J. (1957) An experimental approach to the psychopathology of childhood: encopresis, *Br. J. med. Psychol.* **30**, 146–175.

*8. Woodmansey, A. C. (1967) Emotion and the motions, *Br. J. med. Psychol.* **40**, 207–223.

9. Woodmansey, A. C. (1971) Parent guidance, *Devel. Med. Child Neurol.* **13**, 243–244.

10. Bruch, H. (1941) Obesity in childhood and personality development, *Am. J. Orthopsychiat.* **11**, 467–475.

11. Bruch, H. (1939) Obesity in childhood, *Am. J. Orthopsychiat.* **58**, 457.
    Bruch, H. (1940) Obesity in childhood, *Am. J. Dis. Child.* **59**, 739–781.

12. Millican, F. K. and Lourie, R. S. (1970) The child with pica and his family, in *The Child in his Family* (eds. Anthony, E. J. and Koupernik, C.) Wiley Interscience, New York.

13. Cooper, W. (1957) *Pica*, Charles C. Thomas, Springfield, Illinois.

14. Lourie, M. *et al.* (1963) Why children eat things which are not food, *Children*, **10**, 143.

*15. Morley, M. (1957) *The Development and Disorders of Speech in Childhood*, Livingstone, Edinburgh.
    Pick, T. *et al.* (1967) Perceptual integration in children, in *Advances in Child Development and Behaviour*, p. 192, Academic Press, New York.

16. Reed, G. F. (1963) Elective mutism in children – a reappraisal, *J. Child Psychol. Psychiat.* **4**, 2, 99–107.
    Renfrew, C. and Murphy, K. (eds.) (1964) *The Child who does not Talk*, Heinemann Medical Books, London and the Spastics Society.
    Straugham, J. H. *et al.* (1965) The behavioural treatment of an elective mute, *J. Child Psychol. Psychiat.* **6**, 2, 125–130.

17. Ingram, L. (1963) The association of speech retardation and educational difficulties, *Proc. Roy. Soc. Med.* **56**, 199–203.

18. Andrews, G. and Harris, M. (1964) The syndrome of stuttering, *Clinics in Developmental Medicine No. 17*, The Spastics Society Information Unit, in association with Heinemann Medical Books, London.

19. Boder, E. (1968) Developmental dyslexia, *Claremont Reading Conference, 32nd Yearbook* 173–187.

20. Eisenberg, L. (1966) Reading retardation: psychiatric and sociologic aspects, *Paediatrics*, **37**, 352–365.

21. Advisory Council on Handicapped Children (1972) Children with Specific Reading Difficulties. H.M.S.O., London.

22. Bateman. B. (1966) Learning disorders, *Rev. Educ. Res.* **36**, 1, 93–119.

* Davie, R. *et al.* (1972) *From Birth to Seven*, Longmans, in association with the National Children's Bureau, London.
    Pringle, M. K. *et al.* (1966) *11,000 Seven Year Olds*, Longmans, in association with National Children's Bureau, London.

23. Alberman, P. and Sheridan, M. (1971) Reading retardation, *Devel. Med. Child Neurol.* **139**, 200.

24. Tansley, A. E. and Gulliford, R. (1965) *The Education of Slow Learning Children*, Routledge & Kegan Paul, London.

25. Sheridan, M. D. (1948) *The Child's Hearing for Speech*, Methuen, London.

26. Jensen, A. R. (1969) How much can we boost I.Q. and scholastic achievement? *Harvard Educ. Rev.* **1**, 1–123.

27. Tolstoy, L. (1917) *Anna Karenina*, Penguin Books, Harmondsworth.

## CHAPTER 12

# Psychosomatic Problems

The relationship between body and mind is important in all illness, but is thought to be of particular importance in conditions such as asthma, eczema, gastric ulcer, ulcerative colitis, migraine and rheumatoid arthritis. It is interesting however, that a study into the personality characteristics of patients suffering from a condition throught to be psychosomatic and using patients with fractures in an accident ward as controls, found that the control group has as many personality problems as the groups under study, but the problems were different.

Thus the concept of accident-proneness came about, and indeed many conditions thought to be purely 'somatic' and with a known bacillary causation such as tuberculosis were found to have psychological aspects in respect of course of illness and recovery. Thus the boundaries between the psychosomatic conditions and other illnesses has become less definite. In addition desensitisation following learning theory techniques have been known to 'cure' asthma and we shall see later how fits can be 'cured' by play with the paediatrician. (p. 171).

## A. Factors in Causation

### 1. Genetic vulnerability of target organ or system

Pinkerton (1972) suggests that common to all cases is a basic substrate of vulnerability, which in asthma concerns excessive lability of the bronchial system, in eczema atrophic sensitivity of the skin, and in migraine an anomaly of the intracranial microcirculation to give a few examples.

## 2. The psychosomatic triad

The psychological aspect is multifactorial.

### Personality type and reaction to illness

The very definite personality profiles described in earlier research, such as the driving personality of the peptic ulcer patient, have not been borne out by later studies. Indeed many of the childhood sufferers from asthma, migraine, etc. show a personality which has been described as 'hard driving, anxious to please, compulsive, sensitive'.

Probably personality type is more important in regard to the reaction pattern to stresses and to the particular stress of illness.

### Parental contribution

In this sphere personality factors in the child intermix with the personalities and attitudes of the parents and indeed of the whole family, often complicated by the fact that one or other parent has probably been a sufferer from the same or a similar psychosomatic condition. This parent may overprotect the child, may react by harshness ('I had to suffer it, why not you?') or by a mixture of the two, with the other parent taking the opposing line. The 'sick' child may become a focus for marital tensions, and two-way jealousy situations with siblings are common, the 'well' child envying the invalid his special position and the attention he gets, the 'sick' one envying his sibling the normal life he is able to lead.

Parents may feed into the driving need for success which the child already has and this may activate symptoms.

### Situational stress

This probably has most effect on the actual attacks and the timing of symptoms, pressure at school or home, illness of parents or siblings, anxious anticipation, pleasurable or otherwise, of special events and so on. The autonomic nervous system is involved in triggering off symptoms and reinforcing them.

Nicholas, aged 9, had suffered from asthma since he was 2. His mother had been asthmatic since her early teens, but this ceased after the birth of Nicholas. Mother had an unhappy early life herself having been brought up by her father when her mother died when she was 5 and later by a stepmother from the age of 11 when her asthma started (in order to get attention from father she said).

Nicholas's father died suddenly when he was 9 months old, and mother remarried when he was 2½. He has a stepsister aged 5. Since 2 years Nicholas has been hospitalised frequently for attacks of asthma, for investigation and desensitisation.

At home he is a tense boy, jealous of Sharon. He gets excited about outings, holidays, anything new, so these are kept secret from him. Mother says he can 'bring on' attacks (as she did), so he is commanded to 'stop it' and told to stay in his room till the wheeziness has gone, but sometimes these episodes go on to full-blown attacks and he has to be sent to hospital. A family routine is arranged round Nicholas to 'keep things under control'.

At school Nicholas fits in well, he is keen on sport including football and 'plays whenever he can'. He is 'keeping up academically though absences hold him back'. The headmaster doesn't want to lose him from his school. (I.Q. in the clinic 138, very superior, Reading Quotient 138.)

Mother, stepfather, Nicholas and Sharon were seen individually and for 'family meetings' in the clinic. Mother proved to be manipulative towards all the persons involved in the treatment of Nicholas (paediatrician, headmaster, clinic team) as well as punitive towards him. She attempted to dominate the family meetings and to have the social worker at her beck and call.

Stepfather proved to be a plodding practical man with a 'common sense' approach to Nicholas. He supported mother's attitude, but spent a lot of time with the boy playing football with him, taking him out, etc. Sharon was a pretty, lively, attention-seeking little girl with whom mother appeared to identify.

Nicholas, a serious-looking boy wearing glasses, was a little tense, but with a tremendous sense of humour. His individual sessions were used by him for expression of his very vivid phantasy life, through paintings, clay modelling and puppet play.

## B. Therapeutic Considerations

A global approach is needed aimed at therapeutic improvement by whatever means possible, medical, psychiatric and educational, and the reinforcement of any improvement achieved. It is most important that paediatrician, schoolteachers and clinic team work together to achieve this. This was most important in the case of Nicholas as mother was so manipulative. Children suffering from asthma often do well when taken out of the home situation, but this is not always advisable for other reasons.

## C. Anorexia Nervosa

This is not a truly psychosomatic condition, but is most appropriately included here. It is a fairly rare condition, occurring mainly in adolescent girls and young adult females, but may also occur in boys and young men (less than 1:10).

There is refusal to eat, with amenorrhea, weight loss, secondary anaemia, weakness: about 10 per cent of cases die.

The girl is often immature in both appearance and personality, and non-acceptance of femininity and refusal to grow up is postulated. Adolescent plumpness may be seen as pregnancy possibly by oral impregnation or as an invitation to sexual advances; refusal of food may start allegedly for slimming purposes, but then becomes an end in itself. Sometimes the girl gorges food and then makes herself vomit. She may continue leading a very active physical life for some time and then goes rapidly downhill. The families of these children often function with a facade of normalcy, and faulty interactions tend to be subtle but pervasive. They may need a 'sick' child to preserve family 'happiness'. The girls often have a hostile ambivalent relationship with their mother and in some cases there is an obsessive need to gain control over their bodies.

*Treatment*

Because of the seriousness of the condition, treatment may have to be in hospital, and then either a strict authoritarian regime aiming at getting the patient to eat at all costs, 'babying' the patient, or a regime allowing regression may be used. The condition usually improves in hospital, but rehabilitation and psychotherapy before discharge and a strict follow-up are necessary to prevent the relapses which are common. Family therapy, and treatment of the child at home would seem to be the treatment of choice where possible.

### Further Reading

\*     Daly, P. (1970) *Anorexia Nervosa*, Maudsley Monographs, London.

Graham, P. J. *et al.* (1967) Childhood asthma: a psychosomatic disorder? *Br. J. prev. Soc. Med.* **21**, 78–85.

Holguin, J. and Fenichel, G. (1967) Migraine, *J. Pediat.* **70**, 290–297.

Jones, R. S. (1966) Assessment of respiratory function in the asthmatic child, *Br. Med. J.* **2**, 972–975.

Leigh, D. and Marley, E. (1967) *Bronchial Asthma,* Pergamon Press, Oxford.
Pinkerton, P. (1967) Correlating physiologic with psychodynamic data in the study and management of childhood asthma, *J. psychosomatic Res.* **11,** 1, 11–25.
Pinkerton, P. (1972) The psychosomatic approach in paediatrics, *Br. med. J.* **3,** 462–464.

### PART III

# In the Clinic

*This section discusses kinds of clinics, their staff and their working at a time when the wind of change is blowing strongly. It follows a child and his parents through the early stages of clinic attendance. The 'classical' Child Guidance Approach is outlined.*

---

CHAPTER 13

## Past and Present Arrangements

### A. Historical Overview

The discussions and disagreements which are going on at the present time while plans for future child guidance and child psychiatric services are being formulated have characterised its development during the 40 odd years since child guidance clinics were set up in the United States and in England in the 1920s. Two main questions have emerged and are still at the centre of controversy today; the kind of clinic required and under whose aegis, and the staffing and administration of the clinics.

*Kinds of Clinics*

Here the main division was between those who, like Blacker([1]) considered that the need was for two types of clinics with child psychiatrists or educational psychologists in charge, and those who disagreed. The early clinics had medical directors, but hospital-based clinics were few and did not increase until after the inauguration of the National Health Service in 1948. Clinics based on the community were usually run by local education authorities and these either had a psychologist or a psychiatrist in charge, according to orientation and availability of professional staff. There was considerable unease about the isolation of child psychiatry from medicine, and paediatricians for example began to press for child guidance clinics based on hospitals to forge links between child psychiatrists and paediatricians.

A step forward was the setting up of 'joint clinics' during the 1950s and this has been a continuing trend; with the clinic premises being owned by health (or sometimes education) authorities, who provided most of the professional staff (psychiatric social worker under health and psychologist under education). But since diagnosis and treatment was considered a medical responsibility the child psychiatrist was appointed by the Regional Hospital Board.

Although this arrangement has on the whole worked well, the issue of 'Guidance or treatment'([2]) has continued to be argued, but there has been gradual acceptance that child guidance/psychiatry is a specialist medical service operating under medical directorship. Flexibility and variety however could be seen to have advantages, as pointed out by Kahn.([3])

We may now look at these clinics as they function today.

*Local authority joint clinics*

These are community-based, often operating in buildings in which other health department clinics are carried (providing useful links with health visitors) or in which remedial work is done (providing links with educationalists). They have close links with the schools, through school medical officers,* and also through educational psychologists who may work part-time in the school psychological service; but increasingly with family doctors and with local hospitals. Some child psychiatrists have sessions with paediatricians as part of their contract, and some also work part-time with mentally handicapped children.

*Hospital-based clinics*

These have had close links with family doctors and, of course, paediatricians and other specialists in their own hospitals, and fewer contacts with schools, but have become increasingly aware of their community responsibilities.

*Roles outside clinics*

For some time child psychiatrists have worked in children's homes, remand homes, and approved schools, schools for maladjusted, etc, sometimes free-lance, sometimes as part of their contract.

*Community physicians

## B. Clinic Staff

From the start the 'team approach', as envisaged by Healy in the early 1920s, of psychiatrist, social worker and psychologist, has been utilised in child psychiatry. Warren([4]) comments, 'This procedure, whatever fun has been made of the 'team', is still of fundamental importance and has influenced the practice of psychiatry in general . . . . the 'team' remains a main road to the patient and his family. He also considers that criticisms of the so-called child guidance approach to child psychiatry for rigidity of method 'hardly applies in this country today, where Child Guidance and Child Psychiatric Clinics mostly show a broad approach and tackle problems that would formerly have been excluded'.*

### *Child psychiatrist (Area Health Authority)*

At present as Medical Director([8]) of the clinic his principal responsibility is for every patient referred to the clinic in relation to diagnosis, assessment and treatment.

He also has certain administrative duties connected with allocation of work, keeping of records, confidentiality, etc.

The child psychiatrist also on account of his medical training and knowledge of paediatrics and paediatric neurology, is alert to the possible organic aspects of a case, and he may make a diagnosis himself or refer to the appropriate specialist.

The main part of his work is with the clinic team with the members of whom as far as professional working goes he has equal partnership, with each member of the team complementing the others. The child psychiatrist frequently takes over the treatment of the child 'patient', but in most clinics there is flexibility and he may, in fact, take a part in the treatment of the whole family; he may treat the parent(s) while someone else sees the child, or he may himself, or with his whole team, visit a school or community home to work with the staff there on the treatment of the child. He also has duties and opportunities in regard to teaching and research.

Many child psychiatrists also work in community homes, schools for maladjusted or other special schools.

### *Psychologist*

The director may be a 'clinical psychologist' based on the clinic, visiting schools mainly in connection with cases referred to the clinic, but available at

*See also Harrington,([5]) Hawkey,([6]) and Martin([7]).

those times for general discussion and consultation. Or he may be an 'educational psychologist' part of whose duties will be to visit schools, in a consultative capacity, and he may in fact be based part-time on the schools.

The psychologist is orientated to objective approaches and a considerable part of his work in the clinics is the study of intelligence, and academic attainment which is linked to it. Intelligence tests are devised to test capacity in a variety of ways. The psychologist may also assess personality either by projective techniques (e.g. the 'ink blots' of the Rorschach test) or by the use of questionnaires.

He may also assist in diagnosis in cases of special learning problems or suspected organic damage, where particular techniques such as the Frostig test, the Goldstein tests, or the Bender Gestalt may be used.

A psychologist working in both schools and clinics may have problems in both spheres, but his valued role as a member of the clinic team should minimise any difficulties here. However, in schools his involvement with the clinic team can be an embarrassment to him. One psychologist has written,([9]) 'The best results come when there is awareness of a problem and doubts as to a solution. The worst comes when teachers have no doubt about the previous procedures and prove their point in that other pupils are all right when treated with methods to which this particular child does not respond'. The school may ask the psychologist, 'How can we cure this child's bad behaviour in school?' and if no answer is forthcoming 'the clinic is expected to cure it' (Kahn and Nursten([9])).

Many psychologists take an active part in research.

### Social worker

The specific role of the social worker is with the parents or those who have care of the child, or with the family as a whole. Initial interviewing with parents is aimed at assessment so that interest is focused on the presenting problem, the personal history of the child and the family history, but the search for facts must never be by intrusion or insistence, for the long-term relationship with the parent(s) is more important than the immediate need.

Collection of collateral information and liaison with other individuals and agencies concerned with the child is important. The social worker also assists in administration especially in regard to keeping contact with patients on waiting lists and dealing with appointments.

Through casework she usually takes care of the treatment of the parent(s), or helps in short-term treatment or family treatment. She takes part in teaching as member of the clinic team and also by supervising the work of individual students, and may also engage in research either on her own or with another member of the team.

The social worker has especially close contact with other social agencies interested in the child's welfare and in practical methods of alleviating hardship and suffering.

All or most social workers are interested in welfare, but the social worker who has been specially trained to work in child psychiatric clinics has learnt a particular technique or skill for 'casework.' The caseworker starts with the problem presented by the parents or family, and by assisting their usual modes of adaptation, by 'working through' those past experiences which determine present behaviour, and often by using psycho-analytic concepts to aid understanding helps them to continue to function and perhaps function better in spite of their problems. She understands how resistance and ambivalence may hamper her work with her client; although she does not set out specifically to treat her client by psychoanalysis as the child psychiatrist may. However the boundaries of casework have been extending and training in advanced casework and in techniques of group and family therapy have increased the field of operation of the social worker (Rubinstein and Levitt([10])).

*Psychotherapist*

Many clinics are fortunate in having a psychotherapist, who usually has a degree in psychology and who in addition has worked in a department which offers a theoretical and practical training in communicating with children in on-going therapy.

*Other professional staff*

Working with the team there may also be a remedial teacher, whose premises may be within the clinic building or outside it, and possibly a teacher or therapist in charge of a day centre for maladjusted children.

Speech therapists may have rooms in the same building, and although not part of the clinic team; fruitful discussions and collaboration often take place.

*Clinic secretary*

She is a most important person, and may be thought of as a non-professional member of the clinic team.

She has the direct responsibility for looking after records, for dealing with appointments and keeping a balance between the needs of the families outside referring agencies and people, and the needs of the different members of the clinic team for the time of other members. She keeps tabs on the implementation of plans and details of treatment which are known to her and makes sure that individuals do not 'slip through the net'.

In addition she is often the first and later the most frequent person to be in contact with families and others either by telephone or by personal meeting, and her approach is most important, setting the tone of the clinic approach.

### Bibliography and Further Reading

Items marked * are particularly important sources. Unnumbered references provide alternative sources to the references quoted immediately above.

1.  Blacker, C. P. (1946) *Neurosis and the Mental Health Services,* Oxford Medical Publications, London.
    N.A.M.H. (1965) *Child Guidance and Child Psychiatry as an Integral Part of Community Services,* N.A.M.H., London.
2.  Leading article, 1959, Guidance or treatment. *Br. med. J.* **2,** 1391–1392.
    Leading article, 1961, Trends in child psychiatry, *Br. med. J.* **2,** 1551.
    The report of the committee on Maladjusted Children (1955) (The Underwood Report), H.M.S.O., London.
3.  Kahn, J. H. (1962) The local-authority child-guidance clinic, *Lancet,* i, 959–960.
    *Report of the Committee on Local Authority and Allied Personal Social Services,* (1968) (The Seebohm Report) H.M.S.O., London.
    Royal Medical Psychological Association (1967) Memorandum on the Underwood Report.
*4. Warren, W. (1971) You can never plan the future by the past, *J. Child Psychol. Psychiat.* **11,** 4, 241–257.
5.  Harrington, M. (1960) The integration of child therapy and casework, *J. Child Psychol. Psychiat.* **1,** 2, 113–120.
6.  Hawkey, L. (1968) Collaboration within the therapeutic team, in *Ventures in Professional Cooperation* (ed. Barnes, E.).
7.  Martin, F. and Knight, J. (1962) Joint interviews as part of intake procedure in a child psychiatric clinic, *J. Child Psychol. Psychiat.* **3,** 1, 17–26.
8.  Royal Medical Psychological Association (1961) The Function of the Medical Director of a Child Psychiatric (Child Guidance) Clinic.
9.  Kahn, J. H. and Nursten, J. P. (1968) *Unwillingly to School,* 2nd edn., Pergamon Press, Oxford.
10. Rubinstein, M. and Levitt, P. (1957) Some observations regarding the role of fathers in child psychotherapy, *Bull. Mem. Clinic* **21,** *16.*

# CHAPTER 14

## First Contacts

### A. Referral

The question of 'direct' referrals has been a moot point especially in clinics based on the community. In hospital clinics it rarely arises. Should an individual, e.g. a headteacher or school welfare officer or an organisation such as the Probation or Social Service Department be able to refer a child to the clinic without going through a doctor? It has usually been assumed that referral from the Courts would come directly, perhaps because of the urgency, and certainly in some clinics, departments such as Probation, and the Social Service Department have made direct approaches. If these, why not others — a headteacher or school welfare officer when a child is about to be against open referral is that child psychiatry is a specialist medical service, and that open referral would be confusing and waste scare specialist skills. The family doctor is the key person, and all referrals should be known to him, but may come from school medical officers, paediatricians and other medical persons, who will be consulted by the individual or agency who has recognised the need. It is not often that necessary referrals are 'blocked' by this method, nor should they be delayed. At present there is a move away from this 'medical model'.

Clinics based on the community will tend to receive most referrals from family doctors and Community Physicians, and hospital-based clinics from family doctors and paediatricians.

The referral letter may tell much or little about the problem. It may not even be written by the person who wished for the referral, so it is important to know who really initiated the referral and why. The main sources are the home and the school. We saw in Chapter 10, that parents and teachers often do not see the same child, and that they worry about different aspects of a child's behaviour. This partly explains the misunderstandings and ill feelings which sometimes arise over referrals; but underlying this are deeper reasons and unconscious motivations.

It is easy for parents and teachers to see eye to eye about the need for referral for a clear cut medical or surgical condition and we saw how parents and teachers agreed about problems such as stammering and nailbiting, tics, school refusal and learning problems but diverged on the more subtle and subjective ones. We have seen also that it is rare for the child himself to see a need for referral, far less seek it, and that he is referred because someone is concerned, usually about his behaviour, and wishes it to be changed.

It often appears, in fact, that the child's behaviour threatens the stability of the family and home (or school); in fact that someone is put on the spot by it and by him. It is feared that worse may happen unless 'something is done'.

It is easy to see how the concurrence and the divergence arise. Teachers feel they are falling down on their job if the child fails to attend school or does not work, while parents feel they are failing if their child cannot accept school and do well there. If the child is also a disciplinary problem at school the situation is made worse. Some teachers are able to recognise their feeling of failure and frustration, as some parents can; but very often neither can and each blames the other. It is sad to see a concerned teacher and a devoted mother reach a peak of misunderstanding and distrust, and for the child to be between them.

According to his mother, Roy, aged 7, had always been excessively shy and, fearing he would not settle at primary school, she obtained a post as helper at a private kindergarten on the understanding that Roy would be accepted there. At first Roy could not settle to play or mix with the other children, but mother managed to have him moved to a class where the teacher was more accepting of mother's presence and frequent suggestions. Roy became much more settled and happy, but still looked to mother to do certain things for him and he spoke little, or in a rapid gabble which mother alone could proudly interpret. At home Roy could not remain in the house if mother went out although his father, grandmother or older sister was there. He did not start primary school until he was 5½, but for the first year, with a teacher mother knew, he seemed quite happy. In his next class, however, there were soon problems. Roy made no attempt to learn anything, did not mix with the other children, and if taken outside at playtime merely stood where he had been placed. He never spoke to his teacher, but would ask his headmaster to sit next to him at dinner. The headmaster wrote 'and I usually do'. His class teacher was 'very gifted with children, using a positive approach'. Her own story is important. She was a widow who had brought up four children, one of whom was spastic, but this girl had attended the ordinary school, and had learnt to do everything for herself. Roy, on the other hand, at 7 still expected his mother to put on his coat for him, and she expected to do it. He did not like to be asked to do anything he did not want to do, or perhaps felt he could not do, and his withdrawal seemed to be a response to his teacher's wish to involve him more. The teacher came to the clinic saying 'Please do something about this mother', while mother's parting words were, 'What are you going to do about the teacher?'

## B. Polarisation and Partisanship

When a case such as this is presented at a clinic, people take sides. This may be denied. 'We are scientifically trained people with an objective approach:' is often claimed but I have seen it too often not to recognise it. I have felt it in myself. The most usual thing is for the psychologist to side with the teacher (school) the social worker with the mother (family) and the psychiatrist with the child (patient). Ideally this should not happen, but when it does, if we recognise it for what it is we are less likely to get caught in the tangle.

If the referral is to be seen as helpful, those persons concerned with the child who did not seek it must be involved as fully and as tactfully as possible. The family doctor may resent it since he who has known the family since the mother was a little girl did not think it necessary. The teacher may remark 'We have many children more in need of child psychiatry than this one'. If the parent then explains that at home the child soils and pilfers, the response may be 'Well, that is a home problem then', and among themselves the teachers may agree, 'There's nothing wrong with John, he just needs a new Mum'.

In addition there may be misunderstandings of parental aims, particularly if there is a cultural gap between family and school, perhaps in an immigrant West Indian family, or a family of a low social class. In both cases communication problems, as well as differing aims and aspirations, widen the gap between the family and the school. Some of these aspects were considered in the Halsey Report[1] discussed in Chapter 3.

Headteachers may request referrals without consulting the parents, who have a right to know what is being suggested for their child, while parents may ask that the school (who also feel thay have a right to know) is not told about the referral. They may feel that the school may give a picture of the child which would be damaging. Parents, even more than teachers, are likely to feel threatened by the clinic referral, perhaps misunderstanding its function ('My child is not mentally ill or subnormal.'); or if there has been antisocial behaviour outside the home they may fear the reaction of school or neighbours 'if they know we are coming to the clinic for that'.

Mrs T. did not bring Lawrence to the clinic till a year after he was first referred, and only then because the school said they could not contain him any longer. She was in a panic, 'If only he would do what his teachers and his father tell him to do there would be no need for him to come', she said with tears in her eyes, and for a long time was quite unable to look at her extremely bad relationship with Lawrence.

The child becomes involved in the attitude of the parent and the teacher to the clinic, for the parent projects her doubts onto the child, and insists he would be 'upset' at having to come to see a psychiatrist. It may be suggested that the doctor should visit the home as a 'friend of mother's', and one head of a junior school colluded with the parents by telling the child that he had been specially selected to go to the clinic to do some tests for 'my friend Mr Jones' (the psychologist).

At school the teacher may say 'Do you have to go to the clinic *again*?' or another 'What good does it do anyway? All you do is play'.

## C. Expectations

Some schools and family doctors indicate their lack of expectations in regard to the clinic by referring very few cases, others refer many.

All too often the hope or expectation of parent or teacher is unrealistic; the child has been sent to the clinic because he is too maladjusted to be dealt with by ordinary common sense methods and he is being handed over to the 'experts' to be made over and returned acceptable. The idea of working with the clinic is not commonly present initially, but parents and teachers do want to know what is going on and they frequently look for advice. Teachers are in the worse position. The parents after all, do go to the clinic with the child and should have contact with 'the experts', but the teachers, who have probably gone to a lot of trouble to achieve the referral and in making reports, may feel they are kept out of the picture. If some special understanding of their pupil has been achieved at the clinic they 'should know about it so that they may use it in handling the child'. This is true in the case of exceptionally high or low intelligence or specific learning problems, or some special psychological difficulty such as a phobia about going to the lavatory for fear of contamination, and this sort of information is usually passed on. It may also help the teacher to know that Jeremy, who seems as though he 'couldn't care less' really does care, or that a child who suddenly fails to concentrate is really too anxious to be able to do so at present. But, by and large, specific advice about handling is rarely useful, and often open to misinterpretation. After all, school is school and teachers are teachers, some marvellous, some less than marvellous like people the world over, but on the whole, like mothers, 'good enough'; and it is often sufficient for the teacher to know that the child does have problems and then to use his own intuition and expertise in handling the child rather than adapt someone else's recipe for his use.

## D. First Contacts

Except in the rare cases where the parent makes a direct contact with the clinic perhaps on the advice of a mother who has been attending, the first contact is with the person who initiated the referral and we have seen how important it is that the referral is presented in a positive way with no hint of threat, by someone whom the parent likes and trusts.

Now the family wait to hear from the clinic. Unfortunately most clinics have waiting lists and decisions regarding urgency and priority are among the most difficult which have to be taken in the clinic. In doubtful cases or where there is a need to give some support to the family while they wait for a full assessment, the social worker may telephone, or invite the parent to the clinic, or visit the home. If the referral has come from school the educational psychologist may visit the school for the same reason. If the case does not appear urgent and the waiting period likely to be more than a week or two, a letter may be written explaining the position and suggesting that the parent contact the clinic should the situation deteriorate. In all cases the approach from the clinic must be a concerned and welcoming one. At one clinic where the outgoing mail went through a central office, enclosed with the usual friendly letter inviting the family to the clinic went a printed slip stating, 'If you do not keep this appointment you may be liable to a fine of £5' (J. H. Khan and J. P. Nursten([2])).

The appointment letter is usually addressed to both parents, with the explanation 'We like to see both parents', or it may be suggested that the father should attend a subsequent interview. Some fathers would attend in any case, but in most mother only would come out of tradition especially in working-class families. Home visits have been mentioned: these are used by some clinics as their first contact with the family or at least in the early stages. The undoubted advantage of getting a complete picture of the home in action, of seeing the other children and also perhaps the extended family and neighbours, is offset by the fact that the visitor may be regarded as 'just another busybody', and because it robs the family of the right to reveal matters concerning their home and personal affairs as and when they choose. In certain situations and at a later stage a home visit may be seen as positive and helpful.

### E. First Impressions

The family may be familiar with the clinic building, having visited other departments, or the place may seem strange and rather forbidding. In the past, clinics have often been in large old houses, maybe tucked away in odd corners or attics, but these lend a sort of cosiness absent in hospital psychiatric clinics and presumably absent in purpose-built health centres where many clinics are likely to operate in the future. The oddest rooms may have unexpected advantages. In one clinic my therapy room was a disused cloakroom with a row of washbasins with white tiles and inset mirrors above along one wall. The tiles proved ideal and exciting for finger-painting and games were played with one withdrawn child using the mirrors. The room the children have liked best is a circular one, in a small turret leading from a larger room but with its own door which the children will firmly shut.

Waiting rooms may be a bit austere, and one was simply on a corridor with a peremptory notice 'Child Guidance cases wait on the form'.

We learn quite a lot by the way families wait. In one attic clinic there is a large landing divided by a table with magazines on it, and families have a choice of sitting in full view of people ascending the stairs, or tucking themselves away between the table and a short staircase going up under the sloping roof. Some children press close against mother or father, as though unwilling to be prized off, others sit at the opposite side of the table or even stand reading a comic with their backs to the whole proceedings. Parents may sit close together, or at opposite side of the table; father may hold a newspaper up in front of his face, while mother may take out her knitting or crochet (one mother used to bring a large tapestry on a frame). If there is unavoidable delay, some families wait patiently (one mother waited 2 hours in another part of the building), others go to the office to complain or bang on the doctor's door, if they know which one it is.

## F. Procedure

The classical child guidance team approach, presumably arising from a wish to treat the referred child as a patient in his own right, with his own dignity and importance, sets out to interview parents and child separately. Both sides have a chance to get their point of view across. Each member of the team plays his distinct appropriate and equally important part, and where suitable, the expectation is that parallel treatment of parent and child will be arranged.

This method contrasts sharply with the more flexible family orientated approach now used in intake interviews at many clinics.

We look first at the classical approach, and it is important to do this; because this is where it all began, because it has demonstrated its value and should not be lightly cast aside, and because it may still be the method of choice in some cases, and may be used side by side with the newer methods.

However while considering the different intake methods described, the student may like to keep in mind Ackerman's complaint that there has been a tendency in child psychiatry to 'hypothesize a relationship between a piece of the child and a piece of the parent'.

### Classical procedure

The child is firmly regarded as 'the identified patient', and the parents come to the clinic to talk about their problems with this child. At the initial interview the child may be seen by the psychologist, and the parents by the social worker, and this will indicate to the family that child and parents will go their different ways in the clinic. At the next interview it is likely that the child psychiatrist will see the child and parents separately (unless the patient is an adolescent). This is not always well received; the parents may feel that they should be able to put their case to the doctor. They are accustomed to doing this in medical clinics and may even wish the child to hear what they have to say. They want to set the tone, and also hope that the child will show himself in his true light. With the doctor alone he might 'get away' with something. So the parents may feel cheated, and uneasy, although they have an opportunity to talk with the doctor after he has seen the child.

As not every child needs to be seen by the psychologist, it may be preferable for child and parents to be seen by the two other members of the team before he is called in, and he may be able to use his time more efficiently if he has an idea of the areas of difficulty, or of special aspects such as organic or learning problems. However, this approach may lengthen the assessment period.

In any case the feelings of the parents towards the clinic will be communicated to the child. There may be resentment or anxiety about the referral, and possibly attempts to deny the function of the clinic. Or it may be used as a threat and the doctor presented as the person who will punish the child, 'sort him out' or even send him away. How a child separates from the parent will depend on any problem he may have regarding separation, on the parent's attitude and on the circumstances at the time.

Laura, aged 8, was at loggerheads with mother and could only be 'controlled' by father. She was very jealous of her younger brother, aged 4, for whom mother showed a preference. During the initial interview with both parents and brother present she appeared to form an intense relationship with the therapist, but at the next visit, when the therapist expected her to come with her readily, Laura clung to her mother in floods of tears, and then indicated that she would only go into the playroom if her brother came too. In the playroom her tears ceased immediately, and she turned her back on her brother saying that she had been afraid her mother might abandon her, but she'd never 'leave that baby behind'.

In general children find separating more difficult if both parents come, and even more so if all the family come, and the child the only one to be prized away. If mother lingers over leavetaking, wanting to remove the child's coat at the last minute, or if he sees the parents waiting around, he may find it hard to go, and may also wonder whether his parents will be able to hear what he is saying.

It is a new experience for the child to have someone all to himself and although the test procedures gone through with the psychologist give an atmosphere which is not totally unfamiliar, the session with the 'funny' doctor is probably unlike anything he has known before, but it does set up a potentially therapeutic situation between the two of them.

*Alternative arrangements*

A letter is sent to the parents inviting both of them to bring the 'identified' patient to the clinic. One or both parents may come, and may also bring along other members of the family. These are usually younger pre-school children, but may be an older child who is ill, refusing to go to school or at home for other reasons, perhaps a holiday period. This family group may be seen together by the social worker and the psychiatrist in a room where a sufficient number of chairs are provided and also play materials which may be in the centre or a little to one side. The parents may be told at the outset that they will have an opportunity to talk with the social worker later on leaving the child(ren) with the doctor, or this may be suggested when it seems appropriate as the session proceeds, or the whole first session (usually 1½ hours) may be spent with the whole group together. What the family does is just as important as what the family says, where they sit, whether mother (or father) takes the toddler on her knee, how the children use the play opportunities, do they play together, separately or parallel, do they squabble or compete for attention from parents or from the doctor, who, with the social worker, may utilise the session purely for observation and as part of the assessment, or as the beginning of therapy, talking to the family about what is going on.

Family dynamics are brought quickly into the open, and it is sometimes surprising (see Ackerman([3])) how much can be said by children and accepted by parents even in a first interview.

Mr & Mrs Jones had brought Karen, aged 7½, (identified patient) and also Susie, aged 6, to the clinic. The parents sat down with me in comfortable chairs at one end of the room. Susie took no interest in our talk but went off to play with a farmyard in a distant corner. Karen also played near her with a doll's house but kept coming across, usually leaning against her father. The couple described an argument and Karen looked up and said to her father 'you threw scissors and they stuck in the wall'.

Even if the parents bring only the referred child, the trio may be seen together by social worker and doctor, with the child taking what part she wishes in the group talk, according to age and inclination. What happens may be very revealing.

Christine, aged 8, had been referred for poor progress at school and tantrums at home especially with mother. Mother, father, social worker and I settled in a half-moon shape while Christine went off exploring the play opportunities. She brought over two boxes of 'Playdo'. She took out lumps and gave one to each of us (the largest one to mother) asking us to make something. She pushed a low table so that we could mould on it if we wished. The social worker quickly made a rabbit and a fish, and thus encouraged, father and I made an animal each, mother handled her large piece of dough and gave it back to Christine saying 'That's nice and soft for you'.

Another way, which may be used routinely, or with particular families, possibly those who may find difficulty in keeping up attendance, is to write a letter specifically inviting the whole family to attend, indicating 'this is the way we work at this clinic'. From the initial intake interview a plan may be made, perhaps to go on to 'family therapy', or to some form of 'vector therapy' or to utilise certain members of the family group in the treatment of the referred child, or to plan occasional family meetings in addition to individual sessions, or to arrange meetings with father, either individually, with his wife or in a father's group. The possibilities are many.

## Bibliography and Further Reading

1. Halsey, A. (1972) Educational Priority, H.M.S.O., London.
2. Khan, J. H. and Nursten, J. P. (1968) in Chapter 9 of *Unwillingly to School*, 2nd ed., Pergamon Press, Oxford.
3. Ackerman, N. (1958) Toward an integrative therapy of the family, *Am. J. Psychiat.* **114**, 727–733.
4. Howells, J. (1968) *Theory and Practice of Family Psychiatry*, Oliver & Boyd, Edinburgh.

## CHAPTER 15

# The Assessment Period. Classical Method

## A. Parents' First Interview

The parents have probably already met the psychologist and social worker. Nevertheless the first interview with the psychiatrist has a special importance for them.

However they may feel about the referral they have, for whatever reason, taken the decision to bring their child to the clinic thus initiating a relationship between themselves and the psychiatrist. One or both parents may attend. The husband may come in response to the request or to support his wife, or because he is interested in the clinic findings, especially if educational problems are involved. He may come alone if his wife is ill, inadequate or afraid of the clinic. Some fathers attend every interview; others only at special times.

For the psychiatrist this interview is an opportunity to allow the parents to talk easily and involve themselves personally in what they are saying about their child. As they do so their own feelings, hopes and attitudes about assessment and treatment become apparent, and may indicate unconscious resistance, shown outwardly as scepticism, distortion or gratitude and lack of realism. There is often a fear of psychiatry in general and psychotherapy in particular. This is seen as liable to unleash aggressive or sexual feelings in the child, and they fear that an existing disorder (especially if the child is showing sexual or antisocial behaviour) would be exacerbated. Psychoanalysis they believe is only interested in uncovering 'one thing'. Thus they deny that their child has sexual and aggressive strivings. If the parents have emotional problems themselves their fears and denials are stronger.

From the first they are anxiously involved with the child and with the referral, the more so as they are dimly aware that they are in some way responsible. Initially they may present the child as impossible, difficult (less often odd), and themselves as model parents who have only striven for their child's good. They boast of the things they have done for him and the sacrifices they have made, finding it hard to face their feelings of failure and inadequacy. Their hope may be that the psychiatrist will come up with an answer which confirms their picture of an impossible child whose behaviour requires changing.

They are not really looking for an inner change in the child since they fear the methods which might bring this about. They often have a ready-made solution themselves, a school with a stricter discipline, a boarding school or a move to another district, a sort of geographic cure; or perhaps something physical which would 'explain everything'. They give reasons why they should not come to the clinic, they were not consulted, the child should not miss school, he is already improving and so on. The feelings are complex and partly unconscious, and the reasons rationalisations. To show irritation or to ridicule the suggestions would be to ignore not only the unconscious phantasies but the fact that we are being presented with a whole family problem, and that family interaction may have stabilised itself round the child's disturbance over a long period and that any change (or even worse a cure) would cause an unbalance of forces in the family. This will be taken up again in the section on family therapy, and the student may ask himself whether the family approach is more or less threatening.

The child's problem may be an intermediary between the parents and the psychiatrist. Howells has called the child 'the Ambassador'. The parents' initial attitude to the psychiatrist will probably be a mixture of submission (traditional attitude to the expert) and aggression (defensive), but they may find themselves relaxing when they meet someone who is prepared to listen to them, who is not seeking to air his views, but who is concerned not only with their child but also with them. The danger is that in this situation they may reveal things which they may later regret, that they may become over-cooperative, and that the psychiatrist may accede to their expectation of advice. This places the parents in a dependent (non-parent) position *vis-à-vis* the psychiatrist. Nevertheless the parents need to be told something. They need to hear something about any tests which have been done, the opinion which the team have regarding diagnosis and treatment.

### B. James's First Interview

James, aged 7, had been referred because his father was worried about 'poor progress at his preparatory school', and the family doctor added 'jealousy of younger brother'.

James was a tall, well dressed, good looking boy. Although it was his second visit to the clinic he felt he needed his father to go with him into my room but managed to come alone. He said at once, 'I can't do anything well' and looked around as though he thought I might be going to give him something hard to do. (He was a restless, distractible boy who, from the outset, questioned my role in the clinic and in his life, and who, in the presence of marked anxiety, voiced very clearly the uncertainties many children feel in the clinic situation.) He had brought some school books to show me (he left them behind) and told me about a teacher who wanted to cane him 'but I caned her instead' (phantasy). He looked at me out of the corner of his eye, 'Are you a teacher? Is this a school?' he wanted to know. We went into the playroom in the tower. He studied the paintings and daubs on the walls, 'Is that allowed?', then spilled some sand on the floor. 'Is that allowed?' (testing out). I said that this was a room just for children and me and that we can do more things in it than in most rooms. He became excited, jumping up and down, 'Can I do what I want then, won't you tell me off ever?' I told him that I would not let him hurt himself or me badly or do damage that mattered (limits). He became quiet, then looked round the room again. 'Other children come, will you let me smear their paintings, break up their clay pots?' I told him that I look after their special things and his. He spent the rest of the time wandering around the playroom, in and out of the larger consulting room which also had some playthings in it, anxiously and even suspiciously questioning the use of everything (especially the tape recorder). He was much too disturbed and anxious to be able to play. He made no mention of any member of his family, although glances towards the door suggested that he was concerned about the whereabouts of his father.

## C. Case Conference

The case conference, with the team giving their findings in full, has long been standard clinic practice, but it has been criticised as being too detailed and time consuming. Perhaps it is time to examine the usefulness of the 'grand' case conference with the whole professional staff present (this may involve several social workers and psychologists, remedial teacher, psychotherapist and therapist of maladjusted day centre, psychiatrists not involved with the case, and perhaps a speech therapist.) This will be valuable if students are being trained, as the discussion will be widened as more disciplines are included, but should perhaps be occasional 'treats' rather than regular heavy meals.

Alternatives are for only the staff members concerned with the family to meet, or for each team member to prepare a formulation presenting positive findings and his view of the case.

The conference is held when the diagnostic interviews are complete, and when most reports are available. Points of doubt and difficulty are brought out and plans for further investigations are made. The child and his family are looked at for strengths and weaknesses, and the fit between the child and family, and pathological interactions are discussed. The child's life at school and in the community and his relationships with peers and authority figures is examined.

An attempt is made to differentiate between those factors which can be changed (by medical, educational, social and psychotherapeutic means) such as learning difficulties or emotional disturbance, and those which cannot, such as severe subnormality or brain damage, so that a realistic appraisal can be made of the kind of help required.

A plan for treatment is usually outlined at the conference. This may involve remedial help, environmental changes inside or outside the family. Other agencies may be drawn in (or are already involved) which will bring new influences into the life of child and family.

In a large number of cases some form of help is offered at the clinic. The kind of help, frequency and regularity of interviews, selection of therapist and caseworker vary according to need.

The 'classical' method has been parallel treatment of child and parent, which will be described in some detail, while remembering that a variety of other methods may be employed alongside or instead of the original method.

### D. Explanation to Parent(s)

The parents must be given a part in the decisions, in this case, to say whether they feel they can make a commitment to the clinic, to bring the child and to come themselves. They may question the need for separate treatment, which brings in their own involvement, though often their awareness and acceptance of this develops as treatment proceeds. They need to understand something about the whole business of treatment. With young children they can be told that some children have difficulties in making adjustments, and that it may help them to have an opportunity to work through these problems in a special situation with an objective adult who is not in a position to use the child's disclosures for or against him in any way.

There has to be some way of softening the fact that the child will be confiding in someone other than the parent (very worrying and threatening to the parent who is feeling guilty). It can be explained that since the fears and anxieties which the child has have been built up from experiences with the people who are closest to him, parents, siblings, teachers, etc, he will have had little opportunity to explore and examine his feelings in either the home or the school situation. The child will see the same person at the same time every week if the treatment is to help. The treatment session must be viewed as his own private hour and he must feel completely free to talk to his therapist. For this reason it is essential that the child does not feel any necessity to give an account of the events or conversations that occur.

If the child asks questions he may be told that he will be going each week to see Dr X. in the clinic, and if he presses the parent further that it seems to help children to have someone to do things with and talk to all alone.

Parents will be advised to send the child in old clothes, which won't be spoilt. They may find it hard to accept these suggestions, and in many practical ways it is easy for a parent to sabotage the treatment. She may send him in his 'Sunday best', she may come late, or miss appointments, taking no account of the importance of regularity which has been explained to her. She may make derogatory remarks to the child about the clinic or make a joke of his treatment. All this has to be accepted and worked with.

Or she may expect miracles, only to be disappointed at slow progress, or even worsening of the child's condition. The parent should be prepared for changes in the child during treatment in both directions, and it may be possible to help her to see the difference between alleviation of symptoms and an inner alteration in the feelings of a child so that he becomes happier and therefore a person who fits in better.

### E. Confidentiality

*Conference, open and closed*

The clinic team usually confer privately, but sometimes invite interested persons using the opportunity to make contact with teachers, family doctors, probation officers etc. Alternatively a member of the team (or indeed the whole team in some cases) may visit the school, or children's home. These contacts do much to dispel the alleged mystery about child psychiatry.

However, wherever the contact is made, it is important to respect the confidences which parent and child have given at the clinic. It is often difficult for those genuinely concerned about the child to understand this, especially as they may know or suspect much of what has been divulged. A distinction may be made between 'the open side' where a recommendation can be made regarding educational or medical matters, residential school etc. and 'the closed side' where regular treatment sessions are planned for parent and child. (The same criteria have to be applied to the reading of casenotes.) Naturally the teacher or the person dealing with the child in the children's home would like to be fully involved and share the revelations, and they may rationalise this wish by believing they could do so much more for the child 'if only we know what is really bothering him', but this is not often so, and would be damaging to the child's treatment in the clinic.

## Confidentiality in Treatment*

It is vital that child and parent feel free to reveal themselves as and when they wish and that these confidences are respected. Some aspects will be taken up in the section on treatment. Here it is sufficient to say that it is essential that the child is convinced that his meetings with the therapist really are confidential. He is already worried about what may go on in the clinic, he may have little trust in adults, and he may see the doctor as a powerful figure who will conspire with the parents against him. If the parents seem familiar with the layout and personnel of the clinic he may suspect that they have already talked to the doctor about him, and if his mother sees the doctor alone he feels sure she is making derogatory remarks about him. As the child gradually reveals his private world, which has been secret from those nearest and dearest to him and indeed from himself, he feels exposed and needs reassurance that his confidences will be kept. Therapists may say categorically that they will not tell anyone, ever, or that they will not tell without talking it over with the child first.

## F. James's Case Conference

### Problem

*Referral letter* (from family doctor) 'James's father is worried that after a year at a good prep school he is not learning.'

*Father* (informant) made light of the problem saying that the school were worried, but he was clearly concerned, and revealed that at home James shows excessive jealousy of his younger brother, Rupert aged 4½, and also temper tantrums.

*See Ross.([1])

*Social History* (Social Worker)

*Father.* A slim darkhaired man, wearing glasses. A successful business man, self-employed. His work, social activities partly connected with it, and looking after 'my boys' keep him busy. An only child he was 'a late developer'.

*Mother.* Committed suicide when James was three. An attractive, intelligent girl, she had been a radiographer before marriage. Father described her as unstable 'with an insatiable need for affection. Unfaithful and a pathological liar.' He had been infatuated with her and had married her against his parents' wishes.

She had a depression after the birth of Rupert when James was 2½, became suspicious and possessive, and there were many quarrels with paternal grandparents as she would not allow them to see the children. Rupert was only a baby but James was very sensitive to his mother's moods and used to go tense when she came into the room. Father took over much of the daily care of the boys. Later on mother was admitted to a mental hospital but discharged herself after 6 weeks, and 2 weeks later took an overdose. Father did not take James to the funeral, and the boy did not speak of her until a year later when he asked, 'Has my mother got a grave?'.

*Personal History.* A wanted baby conceived after 2 years of marriage. Normal pregnancy and birth but always difficult and 'highly strung'. Problems over feeding and toilet training. No serious illnesses.

*Rupert, 4½:* 'Just the opposite. Placid and easy going. The clown of the family.' but 'stable' (perhaps implying that James is not).

*Paternal grandparents.* Live in a town 15 miles away. Grandmother domineering, grandfather a bit ineffectual. Keen interest in both boys, 'very concerned' about James's education. Prepared to finance him at public school (where father went).

*Maternal grandparents* keep in touch infrequently, as they live further away. The two sets of grandparents do not get on and father tries to keep them apart.

*Family situation.* Father engaged several *au pair* girls but never had them stay more than 6 months 'in case the boys became fond of them' (and perhaps father too). After one girl left James became very upset, and father decided to be 'mother and father both'. He now has a childless married housekeeper who stays all day and babysits when needed.

*Mrs A.* This housekeeper was also seen by the social worker. A pleasant, kindly, practical young woman, preferring Rupert who she regarded as the underdog. James does not cooperate with her and 'gets round' his father, will not leave him to have his evening meal 'in peace', though Rupert does. James 'bullies Rupert'.

*Mrs B. James's teacher* at an academically orientated traditional preparatory school, also seen. 'Can't understand the boy. He can say clever things when he's in the mood, but will sit for half an hour over one picture sum. In his exam he did three questions, then gave up. One day he can read, the next not a word.' She found him dreamy, chewing his knuckles and sucking his fingers. Once on a nature walk he spoke to her about his dead mother. She told him 'not to brood'.

*The psychologist.* This was James's first experience in the clinic and he found it hard to leave his father who eventually pushed him off. He told the psychologist, 'I'm here because I can't concentrate. I'm at the bottom of the class at school. Here are some of my books. School is hard, no toys and all work' (he looked round the room which contained painting materials, sand tray etc).

His approach to the test situation was tentative and anxious. He hunted for minute discrepancies in each item as though it were a trick not a test. He was so anxious that when counting bricks he forgot what the task was and built a tower instead.

Nevertheless his I.Q. was 130 (very superior). He did not want to read. Read only three words on the card, then gave up. There was no indication of brain damage but some 'scatter' probably due to emotional disturbance.

*Psychiatrist.* (from formulation at interview already described)

An extremely tense boy, frozen into a state of near panic. Has serious problems with learning and with personal relationships. Emotionally at about the 3-year level.

*Discussion* centred first around the nature and severity of James's condition. Was it an anxiety neurosis or was there a developing psychotic state?

James had received spasmodic mothering, and father, because of his own worries about his wife's behaviour, could not give much support to the 'couple', and difficulties over feeding and toileting may have arisen because of this. There was spoiling by both sets of grandparents. James was supplanted by Rupert when he was 2, and initially mother 'took' to Rupert in a way she had not shown with James. However, as she became depressed she became possessive of James, refusing access by the paternal grandparents. He was with her a great deal and father mainly looked after the baby, in whom she had lost interest. At the time of mother's death James was still in a very early stage of development. He had no opportunities to express his grief. He formed a relationship with one *au pair* girl and was upset when she left. His attempts to relate to the housekeeper and to his teacher are unsuccessful (but he is still making them). There did not seem any evidence of perinatal damage. No illnesses. Father had problems when he was young, and there were continued pressures especially from maternal grandmother.

The opinion was that some hereditary instability may exist, but the effect of James's contact with his mentally-ill mother, the father's concern about his instability and the role of the paternal grandparents are probably more important.

The diagnosis was anxiety state, with a tendency to panic and 'shut off', but with no true withdrawal. He was not psychotic nor affectionless, was still working out his feelings in his relationships with father, Rupert and Mrs A, and able to begin a relationship with me and bring some of his feelings out into the open.

## Treatment

*James..* Weekly sessions with the psychiatrist (it was considered that a female therapist was suitable). A period of at least a year was envisaged.

*Father.* Weekly sessions with a mature female social worker, to help him to understand and accept what we are attempting to do with James, and the effect it might have on behaviour, and perhaps a need for mourning; that improvement at school should not be the first aim. It was expected that father would show resistance to any attempt to help him directly but that this might develop later.

## Environmental changes

We all felt that a change of school to a more creative and permissive one with remedial help was indicated, but that it would be unwise to suggest this immediately.

Father did, in fact, make a major change, as he remarried after about 6 months' attendance, and this affected the treatment situation.

## Bibliography

1.   Ross, A. (1958) Confidentiality in child guidance treatment, *Mental Hygiene*, **42**, 60–66.

### PART IV

# Treatment of Child as Identified Patient

*This section deals with certain aspects of the child's treatment in detail. It is assumed that the parent(s) will also be receiving help. In the past it has usually been the mother who has attended for regular sessions with the social worker, but there has been increasing interest in involving fathers in combined treatment as well as in groups of various kinds and in family therapies.*

---

## CHAPTER 16

## Aspects of Psychotherapy

There are two broad approaches to treatment, psychotherapeutic and behaviourist, and the factors which determine choice of treatment for the individual child are the orientation, training and availability of the clinic staff, and the suitability of the child for treatment.

Behaviour therapy has been described in Chapter 2 and appears again throughout the book. In the past the two schools of therapy have kept rigidly apart, publishing their work in different journals, discussing it at different meetings and never recognising that each had something to borrow from the other (and did borrow). Now, although some leading protagonists remain totally critical of the other school, on the whole, and especially in training institutes, there has been a welcome change in the direction of increased understanding and sharing. This is especially so in the sphere of family therapy and this will be reflected in the appropriate section. In addition we have to recognise that learning therapy methods are used in a number of situations in the clinic even when this is not openly recognised.

*Psychotherapy*

This section, however, deals particularly with psychotherapeutic methods, which include psychoanalysis proper, those methods which borrow from it, including non-directive therapy, and some kinds of supportive therapy. Many social work students have asked me for clarification of the writings of leading child psychotherapists, which they have sometimes found confusing, and have wanted to know something about the treatment of individual children, and of 'the secrets of the therapy room'. This opportunity is lacking except in departments where two-way screens provide opportunities for observation and sharing in child therapy.

In psychotherapy the aim is to allow the child free expression of his feelings in a situation where the therapist gives up the right to be an all-knowing adult, where he shows interest in the child, and listens to him and tries to enter his world. In addition the therapist may help the child to correct misunderstandings about his environment, and to develop insight. Insight is recognition accompanied by feeling, and is greater than intellectual understanding, which could result from statements, exhortations or authoritative interpretations by the therapist. Play (Ch. 17) includes all communications between the child and the therapist (Winnicott[18]).

*Schools of psychotherapy*

It is not possible to represent all the major schools of child psychotherapy, so in order to give richness but also diversity I have selected A. Freud, M. Klein and D. Winnicott from this country and V. Axline from the USA. The necessarily brief accounts are likely to do less than justice to the therapists, and students interested in this aspect are advised to seek out their original writings.

## A. Diagnostic Evaluation and Selection of Cases for Psychotherapy

We have seen that symptoms are not a sure guide to diagnosis or need, for the same symptom may receive a different evaluation from teachers and parents and may also have different meanings. Some 'symptoms' may be part of a normal variation, what S. Freud[1] called 'Phase-bound difficulties. The neuroses of childhood are in the nature of regular episodes in a child's development or self-limiting adaptation reactions occurring at periods of stress.' Psychotherapy may not be required for the child though some kind of help may be needed by the parent.

*Personality assessment*

This is a 'structural evaluation' which looks at the integration and development of the child's personality. It has been much used by the psychoanalytic schools and the use of their terms gives a precise meaning to what is being described (Freud A.([2, 3])). Three aspects are studied.

1. The child's psychosexual development. Is it appropriate to the child's chronological age? Has the 3-year-old, for instance, relinquished in the main the baby stage of dependency and insatiable desires? Has the 'libido' moved on or has it remained static?
2. Has the child been able to achieve the separation-individuation appropriate to his age? Has he achieved some autonomy and adjustment to external reality? Have his thoughts and emotions remained archaic while physical and intellectual development have forged ahead?
3. Are defence mechanisms being used excessively or in a rigid way?

### B. The Views of Anna Freud and Melanie Klein*

A. Freud considers childhood neurosis to be due to imbalance between the forces within the personality structure whereby the ego, which should remain fluid and act as mediator between the id and the superego, becomes 'calcified'. The ego may present as either weak or strong, but in either case is rigid and inflexible.([4, 5]) Another aspect of the failure in ego functioning is an extensive and prolonged use of defence mechanisms in an attempt to adapt to reality. A. Freud keeps the child's real situation very much in the forefront and considers the presence of the parents in his everyday life vital. In therapy she aims at undoing repression, mediating between the ego and both the id and superego and replacing the primitive superego with one which is less tyrannical and more in tune with reality.

M. Klein([6]) on the other hand sees childhood neurosis as being due to a massive repression of phantasy due to 'the load of guilt and depression' which affect many aspects of the child's life. It may appear as sleep disturbances (difficulty in getting to sleep, early waking, nightmares and night terrors) problems of feeding and elimination, but also inhibition of intellectual and emotional life. There may be either maladjustment or over-adjustment to educational requirements, inability to learn, play or be creative, intolerance or frustration, and abnormal attitudes to gifts. The importance given by

*Segal gives a clear summary([12])

M. Klein([7]) to these disturbances in the child's everyday functioning is in contrast to her almost total lack of concern for what is happening to the child each day, his parents and their possible psychopathy, environmental problems, etc. She is interested in the child's phantasy rather than reality. Her treatment aim therefore is to liberate the child from the burden of his phantasy life and the anxiety it carries and to free the libido for new attachments (cathexes). She does not intervene if she considers that the child can do this for himself.

Although infantile neurosis has been the main indication for therapy, A. Freud([8]) in particular has also been concerned about children who have developed a deficiency illness (from her wartime nursery observations) and also for those where parental pathology is gross.

## C. Child Therapy Different from Adult Therapy

### 1. Free association

This, the 'fundamental rule' of psychoanalysis means that everything which comes into the patient's mind must be expressed in order to reveal unconscious materials. Young children do, of course, freely associate, as their frequent interruptions when something in a conversation reminds them of something else indicates, but they have a difficulty in using this form of verbal communication in a complete way on request.

Initially this is also hampered by the fact that the child comes to the therapist as a patient but without the wish for treatment which is normally present to some degree in the adult. He is too immature and inexperienced to realise that his feelings or difficulties relate in any way to illness, for they bear little resemblance to illnesses he has had when a 'real' doctor with his pills or medicine made him 'better'. If getting better has any meaning to him it will have to do with having to adjust to unpalatable reality and adult demands. He may have a dim awareness of worry or anxiety, that he is doing things he doesn't want to do and that he doesn't understand such as stealing or wetting the bed, or even that his total life situation is intolerable, but he does not see the doctor as his saviour. He feels no bond with him, and places no confidence in him, at least in the beginning. Because of his immaturity his phantasies may be primitive and magical, he may fear the doctor will try to read his mind or take it away from him or operate on his brain. He is further threatened by seeing everything as white or black, good or bad; his own anger and bad behaviour as bad and himself condemned. If he has been 'in trouble' or threatened with the clinic, therapy as a whole and invitations to 'say everything that comes into your head' or interpretations, may feed into his belief that someone is trying to prove he's crazy, or into his self criticism.

## 2. The 'neutral' role of the therapist

M. Klein[7] considers that as in therapy with adults the child analyst's role is 'only to analyse without a wish to mould or direct. To interpret every aspect of the child's behaviour and play, then calmly wait for the release of phantasy.'

A. Freud sees the analyst as a new object to be used by the child hungry for new experiences, and wishing to complete his development. The therapist carries a responsibility to mediate in the personality dynamics perhaps to curb the id or bolster the superego, but also to offer himself 'for the duration of the analysis' as a model for a superego which will be closer to reality.

Although seeking the release of repression A. Freud[9] expresses a fear that without guidance the drives could seek direct gratification (in action) or become fixed at a particular pleasure point. This has coloured her attitude to permissiveness in the treatment situation.

In later years she has modified these views somewhat, particularly in regard to the stress laid on the educative and retraining role of the analyst.

## 3. Transference

The other cornerstone of adult psychotherapy is the transference situation, which has been defined as 'the attitudes, feelings and phantasies which a patient experiences with regard to his doctor, many of them arising seemingly irrationally from his own unconscious needs and psychological conflicts rather than from the actual circumstances of his relationship with his doctor.' Clearly the more the therapist reveals himself the less he can be a 'blank screen' available for projections.

It is assumed that transference material comes from childhood relationships, but our patient is still a child, and the parents are present and active in his everyday life; he is dependent on them for every satisfaction and gratification real and imaginary. A. Freud[10] considers that since the conflictual objects are still external to the child and not internalised as in the adult transference cannot develop, and that the presence of the real parents in the situation prevents the child from reproducing the situation elsewhere, though he may look to the therapist for what he feels deprived of in the real situation.

M. Klein,([11]) who allows little importance to real parents or real happenings, postulates an internalised 'imago' of both parents, considers that a kind of transference is possible and that the child's relationship with his therapist is entirely one of unconscious phantasy.

### 4. Changes in life situation

An adult receiving psychotherapy, either individual or group, is advised not to make major changes in his life, for example, not to marry or divorce or change jobs while the treatment is in progress. The child patient can make no such promise, James's father remarried while James was undergoing treatment and many other children change schools, have a new sibling, or move house during treatment.

### 5. Permissiveness and limits

All child therapists claim to be permissive but define permissiveness differently. Some consider that all behaviour must be allowed without censure or restraint, others accept feelings, phantasies, thoughts and wishes but discourage or prevent direct 'acting out'.* Most therapists agree that limits should be minimal; that they should be set as and when the need arises. Most therapists find that acceptance of the child's feelings is enough.

However, some therapists claim that 'limits are therapy'. Bixler([13]) may remove the child from the playroom, or transfer him to a group so that limits may be conveyed by the groupmates, but Dorfman counters, 'limits are to protect the fragile therapist', and that reasons given for their use, such as that limits are ego strengthening, limits help the therapist to remain accepting, and that they relieve the child of excessive guilt, are merely rationalisations.

### 6. Counter-transference

This has to do with the feelings which develop in the therapist towards the

*'Acting out' is a term borrowed from psychoanalysis where it applies to feelings aroused in the child during therapy, and properly belongs to the 'transference', but which are 'acted out' in the child's real life. Thus during therapy the child's behaviour may show various changes. The term is also used, widely but loosely (see p. 75) for the child who has not been able to build up an apparatus for controlling libidinal and aggressive feelings, and who 'acts out' in real life those feelings which in our society are kept for thoughts, phantasies and dreams.

child. They relate to feelings or unresolved conflicts which he may have towards his own childhood. The 'good' therapist may be tempted to identify with the child, to seek to become a parent to him, rescuing him from his own 'wicked' parents. Since most therapists will have undergone personal analysis they should be aware of such dangers.

Some therapists bring the counter-transference into the open. Winnicott([14]) and Colm,([15]) though very different in other ways, share rather similar concepts. Winnicott([14]) thought of a 'centre area' in treatment which is inviolable, and a fringe area where spontaneity and intuition can be tried out fearlessly, while Colm in revealing his 'side of the field' and his response to the outer 'defensive me' of the child, shows that he still cares for the 'centre real me'.

### D. Views of Donald Winnicott

Winnicott was a paediatrician for many years, and then went on to become a child analyst.([16,17]) His interest in the child's play and its relation to trust was always a feature of his consultative technique. He cites a case of a girl just over a year old who had been having typical *grand mal* convulsions, as many as five a day, from the age of 9 months. She was also irritable and unhappy. She could not play. Winnicott allowed trust to develop by having her on his knee for periods of half an hour, allowing her to bite his knuckles and throw his spatulas on the floor. After several of these sessions the baby was able 'to enjoy play' and following this she had no more fits and was 'a different child'. Winnicott was closest to M. Klein especially regarding the importance of phantasy but criticised her (and other child analysts) in that she was concerned only with the use of play. He wrote([18]) 'The therapist is reaching for the child's communication and knows that the child does not usually possess the command of language that can convey the infinite subtleties that are to be found in play by those who seek,' and went on 'the psychoanalyst has been too busy using play content to look at the playing child, and to write about playing as a thing in itself.'

Also he had little use for interpretations, especially those he called 'clever', or which were used for indoctrination or to produce compliance.([19]) Interpretations were only of value if they arose when the child and therapist are truly 'playing together', and arose out of 'the richness of the material'. He went even further 'the significant moment is when the child surprises himself'. (This is very different from the control exercised by most analysts over the therapy situation).

## E. Views of Virginia Axline

Axline[20,21] with her child-centred (reflexive, non-directive) therapy follows naturally from Winnicott. Basic to her approach is the idea that the parent(s) and later others, have rejected some part of the child but the therapist must accept all of him.

1. The therapist accepts the child just as he is. He shows a warm friendly attitude so that a good rapport is quickly developed, the child responds to an atmosphere of permissiveness and feels able to express his feelings completely.

2. The therapist is alert to the feelings behind the content and reflects them back to the child. From this (not from interpretations) the child gains insight.

3. The therapist follows rather than leads, respects the child's choices and his ability to solve his own problems if given a chance.

4. The child's immediate responses and capacity to express feelings are the centre of the therapist's interest (feelings are stressed throughout rather than content) and he supplies unlimited support to the child in his efforts to deal with his new experience.

5. Therapy is seen as a period of self testing and discovery with a beginning and an end.

6. The child is not hurried and limitations (such as time limits) are used solely to anchor the child to the world of reality and to stress the responsibility in the relationship. (Axline is not worried about limits, considering that recognition of the child's feelings usually prevents damage. She would even allow limits to be broken, saying 'You wanted to do that', or 'You wanted to show me it was important for you to do that' and only uses physical restraint if serious harm could result.)

To indicate to the child his ability to lead in treatment, Axline uses his words or symbols. If the playing child comments 'the boy did it,' she reflects the word 'boy' rather than saying 'You did it'. If the child questions the therapist's private life she follows 'How would you like it to be?' or if he seeks confirmation for the rightness of some action with conventional standards such as spelling she says 'Here you spell the way you want to' or if he reacts to breaking a toy 'Toys sometimes get broken'.

Such limits as there are, are stated in this same impersonal way. 'Toys stay in the playroom. Time is up for today,' so that in every situation it is the child's feelings which count.

## Bibliography and Further Reading

Items marked * are particularly important sources. Unnumbered references provide alternative sources to the reference quoted immediately above.

1. Freud, S. (1937) *Analysis Terminable and Interminable,* standard edition **22,** 178, Hogarth Press, London.
 * Freud, A. (1946) *The Ego and the Mechanisms of Defence,* International Universities Press, New York.
 *2. Freud, A. (1962) Assessment of childhood disturbances, *Psychoanal. Study Child* **17,** 149–158.
3. Freud, A. (1965) *Normality and Pathology in Childhood,* Hogarth Press, London.
4. Freud, A. (1945) Indications for child analysis, *Psychoanal. Study Child* **1,** 127–149.
 *5. Freud, A. (1968) Indications and contraindications for child analysis, *Psychoanal. Study Child* **23,** 37–46.
6. Klein, M. (1948) Infant analysis, in *Contributions to Psychoanalysis,* Hogarth Press, London.
 *7. Klein, M. (1949) *The Psychoanalysis of Children,* Hogarth Press, London.
8. Burlingham, D. and Freud, A. (1944) *Infants without Families,* International Universities Press, New York.
9. Freud, A. (1928) *Introduction to the technique of Child Analysis, Nervous and Mental Disease Monograph Series,* **48,** New York.
10. Freud, A. (1945) *The Psychoanalytical Treatment of Children,* Hogarth Press, London.
11. Klein, M. (1961) *Narrative of a Child Analysis,* Hogarth Press, London.
12. Segal, H. (1964) *Introduction to the Work of Melanie Klein,* Heinemann, London.
13. Bixler, R. (1949) Limits are therapy, *J. consult. Psychol.* **13,** 1–11.
 * Allen, F. (1942) *Psychotherapy with Children,* Norton, New York.
14. Winnicott, D. W. (1971) *Playing and Reality,* Tavistock Publications, London.
 Smollen, E. (1959) Non-verbal aspects of play in children, *Am. J. Psychiat.* **13,** 872.
15. Colm, H. (1964) A field-theory approach to transference and its particular application to children, in *Child Psychotherapy* (ed. Haworth, M.) Basic Books, New York.
16. Winnicott, D. W. (1941) The observation of infants in a set situation, in *Collected Papers* (1958), Tavistock Publications, London.
17. Winnicott, D. W. (1948) Paediatrics and psychiatry in *Collected Papers* (1958), Tavistock Publications, London.
18. Winnicott, D. W. (1968) Playing: its theoretical status in the clinical situation, *Int. J. Psychoanal.* **49,** 4, 591–599.
19. Winnicott, D. W. (1971) *Therapeutic Consultations in Child Psychiatry,* Hogarth Press and the Institute of Psychoanalysis, London.
 *20. Axline, V. (1964) Non-directive therapy, in *Child Psychotherapy* (ed. Howarth, M.) Basic Books, New York.
21. Axline, V. (1947) *Play Therapy: The Inner Dynamics of Childhood,* Houghton Mifflin, Boston.
 Axline, V. (1964) *Dibs: in Search of Self,* Penguin Books.
 Ginott, H. (1961) *Group Psychotherapy with Children,* McGraw-Hill, London.

## CHAPTER 17

# Play and the Therapeutic Alliance

## A. Play in a Natural Situation

Both S. Isaacs,([1]) who defined play as 'the child's work' and M. Lowenfeld([2]) who included in play 'all activities of the child that are spontaneous and self generating' seemed to be saying that play had a natural value as well as a therapeutic one.

Play to every child who is able to play brings satisfactions which are many and varied; physical contact may bring sensual pleasures involving taste, smell and hearing. Children who have missed out in opportunities to explore their surroundings or to play, not only where parents are rejecting but where they are restricting, with too much emphasis on playpens and cots, may develop a sort of cramped control with loss of spontaneity and poorly developed object relations. These children can expand by exploration both sensory and spatial and here play can be thought of as a therapeutic nurturing agent. This is a primitive kind of play following the pleasure principle.

Later imaginative constructional and creative activity helps the child to understand the social world in relation to himself.

## B. The Materials of Play

*The 'basics', water, sand, 'plastics', food*

These satisfy immature oral and tactile pleasures and are an outlet for aggression or regression but also have special qualities.

*Water* has a neutral quality, it is fluid, things can float, sink or swim in it, it cleans but can be made dirty, can be squirted, poured and drunk. It can be mixed with paint, sand and other things. It can be used passively or aggressively, for control or mastery.

*Sand* is malleable, stable, supportive or shifting, consistency can be varied by the addition of water. When dry it can be sprinkled, when wet it can be moulded, thrown (some adheres), has some of the phantasy qualities of the following

*Plastics.* Clay, plasticine, mud, dough, etc. They allow constant change; can be rolled, kneaded, pounded, joined, separated, made broken and made again. Can be made into figures (this helps with body image and object relations) but can also invest the world with reality and be seen as food or faeces and become invested with phantasy. The changing quality allows for the expression of very aggressive or regressive feelings without danger.

Finger paints form a bridge between plastics and painting.

### Drawing and painting

These may not immediately be used as creative play. Initially the influence of school and television may be too strong, for example a child may start with a conventional house with closed doors, and may not be ready to open the doors, but once the productions are truly free the child is using his own language. Certain devices such as painting on a fold of paper so that coloured blots form when the paper is closed becomes a kind of projective technique, and to some extent so do Winnicott's 'squiggles'.

A child may paint at each session and as therapy proceeds he may use symbols as in fairy tales (the princess, the witch, etc.) or more primitive ones (the sun for father, the moon for mother). Or, primitive again, the child may interpret the drawings in an animistic way, 'an angry mountain', 'a frightened tree', and he may identify with these or with powerful symbols, stars, giants, animals, (but at the same time feel frightened). Often there is over-determination of certain meaningful details such as an extra digit, missing or maimed parts or the gigantic size of a foot or weapon in a picture where everything else is in proportion. Or there may be condensation as in a dream so that the picture represents different aspects of the child or of his memories. Such a picture may be very close to a dream and the child may go on to describe a dream he has had.

The child may depict his own problem. David, an encopretic boy of 6, told me he was in hospital because 'there's something wrong with my tummy'. I asked him to draw it. He drew a house with tiny windows round the edge and the central part empty. Into this space he put 'a person' with two eyes, a round body, at the lower end of the body he drew 'legs' turning them into 'a gate'. 'It's shut. Things can't get out.' Then (overdetermination) he drew a long curly thing 'a tail' with a fish and a piece of meat inside 'They can't get out either'. He had not finished but seized another piece of paper and drew 'another person' with spikes all round inside a big oval, 'It's a hedgehog. It's prickles are all out. It can't get out because the prickles would hurt.' I spoke for the first time. 'Are the prickles always out?' 'When the person sits they are,' said David who had problems passing a stool on the lavatory but who would do it when playing much to the annoyance of his mother.

## Puppetry

Simple glove puppets are best, soft animals encourage regressive and aggressive play, otherwise types rather than actual people (and especially not television characters) are good. But Punch or a monkey representing strong infantile desires, a crocodile oral activities, a policeman the superego or reality, the fairy (good mother) the witch (bad mother) are possible representations.

Play here, as with the plastics, can be very aggressive, but with the possibility of coming alive again. It is more real than clay however, and may be frightening. The child can both identify with the puppet figures but also project onto them.

## Dolls house and figures, world material

These are still more real, some children find them too close to reality and play ceases after the scene has been set, or the child fails to personalise the figures. Personalisation of animals, cowboys and indians or even cars may be less threatening.

*Dressing up and role playing* may be chosen by some children, with expression of phantasies and free verbalizations.

## Materials for regressive play

Food, mentioned under the basics, biscuits, sweets, feeding bottles filled with juice may be left around or available on request. Its presentation may be seen as the therapist giving himself as a good nurturing agent, or as an invitation to regression. The child may react by refusal, gorging, sharing or by regression.

Cushions, rugs, big boxes, balsa wood blocks may also be available and all these may be useful where the aim is to set up a special situation for a child or group of children, but most children needing to regress in therapy will find a corner where they can curl up with a puppet or a baby's bottle or some pieces of cloth to make a nest under a low table.

## C. Play in Therapy (M. Klein, A. Freud, D. Winnicott)

It has been said that because of the pleasure which children have in play that 'play is the carrot which enables the child to continue with the treatment', and Lowenfeld wrote that 'toys to children are like culinary implements to the kitchen. It is what the cook does with them that counts.' Play in the presence of the therapist takes on a special quality and the use made of it by the therapist is vital to the progress of the treatment.

However, play may be used in different ways. Some see it mainly as an observational technique, such as Bender and Schilder who considered play as experimentation with the nature and property of things, and to some degree Lowenfeld who carefully recorded world games using special 'world' material by which the child revealed his emotional and mental state, the emphasis being on reality forms rather than interpretation and symbols.

Although M. Klein([3]) also used a special set of world material toys, the use she made of it is entirely different. The toys are regarded as already having a socialised and symbolic meaning and the child's play with them is regarded almost as a replacement for free association, with each play activity having a symbolic meaning. Each child keeps his own set of toys in a special drawer so that if a child breaks or damages a toy representing, for example, a sibling the therapist can watch what the child does with that toy. Sometimes the child 'loses' it only to find it later, or may deny that this toy was his, or his behaviour with the damaged toy may indicate that he was the attacked toy.

Klein([4]) starts straight in with her therapy without preliminaries; from her reactions the child realises that there is a part of his mind which is so far unknown to him, that his play has a meaning and moreover that this meaning is understood by the therapist. This arouses anxiety which is swiftly dealt with by the therapist who makes an immediate interpretation. The relief which the child feels encourages a further release of phantasy. He comes to realise that the anxiety he feels in the present play situation has to do with happenings in his past, and his behaviour towards the therapist such as cessation of play, blocking, anger, etc. is traced to earlier situations (transference). With gradual removal of resistances deeper and deeper layers of phantasy are reached and Klein claims that as anxiety is relieved the child is free to find new outlets for his feelings, and that the lightening of the load which stems from his communication with the therapist gives him a true wish to continue the treatment. Klein([3]) welcomes great freedom in play and encourages aggressive phantasies and verbal attacks, but she does admit that some psychotic children become difficult to control. She lays great stress on verbalisations. She also uses make-believe games which readily provoke the verbalisations which she considers important to speed the analysis.

A. Freud[5] on the other hand encourages free verbalisations but thinks that free play might lead to release of aggressive trends and that 'the aggression liberated initially by analytic permissiveness may later have to be controlled by the analyst.' She also casts some doubt on the reliability of interpreting symbolic material, and relies on the interpretation of drawings and dreams. She considers the initial period important and originally used it to make herself indispensible to the child by showing interest in him and also a certain power, breaking down his resistances and helping him to become aware of the need to solve certain difficulties. Later she began to use this early period of therapy to interpret ego defences which form a barrier to treatment. She is particularly interested in defences against affects; the child may protect himself by 'acting out' (which may also bring him satisfaction and attention) or he may deny his sad feelings and show instead gaiety, clowning and laughing, or he may show a tender protective attitude to a figure representing a hated sibling; she helps him to see that these false feelings are a defence against true feelings.

A. Freud's therapy is much more 'real', she draws on happenings in his real life, and considers that although the therapist allows hostile phantasies to be projected on to her she also represents the real world, and the child is kept constantly aware of the difference between the world of the therapeutic hour and the real world.

She considers that once the initial resistance has passed, the child's urge towards maturation, his pleasure in play and his relationship with the therapist helps him to continue with therapy while the strengthening of ego functions leads to improved relationships for him outside therapy.

Winnicott wrote 'The natural thing is playing, it is the playing facilitates growth, playing leads to group relations and therefore health. Psychoanalysis has been developed as a highly specialized form of playing in the service of communication with oneself and others.'

Winnicott[6,7] regarded play as a development from transitional phenomena, but shared playing (as in therapy) implies trust and if this has not existed in the original 'shared space' it cannot happen later. When trust is there psychotherapeutic play can take place in the overlapping areas between the child and therapist. Where the child cannot play a means has to be found to bring the child to the point where he can begin to play. This Winnicott was able to do in the case of the baby (see p. 173), and presumably the mother was able to take over there as there was no relapse.

Winnicott([6]) was interested not in the content but in the playing child, and described a 'near-withdrawal state' when the child 'inhabits an area that cannot easily be left', and into which he draws objects from external reality which he uses 'in the service of some sample derived from inner or personal reality'. This produces a precarious balance for the child and the connection between play and bodily excitements adds to this and offsets the pleasurable aspects of play. Play in the presence of and with the therapist takes on a new and shared quality. Winnicott's therapy was certainly child-centred and mainly non-directive, but he did allow himself participation (as in his 'squiggle' games and in his intuitive interpretations).

### D. Children who Cannot Play

Many clinicians have described children who, because of a lack of 'primary experiences', have not advanced far enough emotionally to become neurotic. Aspects of their handicap are that they have not been able to individuate, have not formed object relations or found transitional phenomena, and finally cannot play, phantasise or be creative. In Kleinian terms they have not achieved the depressive position. They may show a symbiotic state, or they may merge with their environment in a way which has nothing to do with adaptation to reality.

Winnicott([8]) wrote, 'Being precedes doing' (but these children have never known the feeling of 'being me') and also that 'relating precedes using', (but these children have never had the experience of relating in an ambivalent way).

Winnicott goes on to describe how they may set up a whole 'false self', which is accepted as the real person, or two selves, one the 'caretaker self', which is taken as the whole person, and a 'little self' which is tiny but more real and healthy.

Such children have been called affectionless, unintegrated, borderline or frozen, and each descriptive term has a value. Dorothy Burlingham and Anna Freud,([9]) who came across numbers of these children in her wartime nurseries, and Winnicott have been among the therapists interested in finding a way to help them. Whereas Anna Freud merely states that psychoanalysis cannot help them, Winnicott([8]) wrote, 'When play is not possible, then the work done by the therapist is directed towards bringing the patient from a state of not being able to play into a state of being able to play'. Barbara Dockar-Drysdale([10]) has developed some of Winnicott's ideas for the treatment of 'frozen' and other emotionally deprived children, and has set up and supervised special treatment facilities in her school and in other establishments. The main needs are nurturing experiences, opportunities for regression, opportunities for narcissistic and pre-oedipal play. It is essential that the institution is able to 'contain' the child during treatment. Others, like Hickin,([11]) have worked out methods for treating deprived children in groups in children's homes.

## E. Latency Period Play and Therapy

We have seen that sexual drives continue to be strong during the years from 6 to 12; also that the child is attempting to fit into the pattern of the culture around him. Where emotional growth and integration have not kept pace with cultural adaptation, fitting in may be too difficult. Frightening phantasies of omnipotence or of attack coming from deeper layers may be very disturbing. In these circumstances therapy which aims at helping may be seen by the child as a threat, since it seems to attack his efforts at coping and control, at his reliance on defence mechanisms, and his attempts to achieve a stronger self image.

Yet at the same time the child can use the therapist to establish reality more firmly and to differentiate clearly between phantasy and reality. Phantasy is often repressed in middle childhood yet at the same time many childhood games have a background of phantasy although rooted in reality and the therapist may make use of this, and the child may be reached in therapy directly through phantasy.

The therapist must tread carefully, accepting and sharing the child's phantasies without fear, and with feeling, empathising with the child through the world of phantasy, which will change as the treatment progresses. At the same time he must remain adult, and rooted in reality.

Many kinds of play, puppets, dressing up, and creative activities are often seen, the child weaving phantasy out of any material, a pencil and paper as in Winnicott's 'squiggles', a piece of cloth, or the memory of a dream. If the games which develop during therapy are too realistic, therapy is blocked, as they do not allow for phantasy digressions, but if they are too rich in phantasy, the child may become too anxious to continue. Such games also do not allow for identification on a reality level.

In middle childhood the child has difficulty also in revealing himself and his feelings towards his parents and substitute adults. This defensiveness is connected with the developmental necessities of these years, and the therapist may have to find a way of combating this when the child refuses to play or to move into any of the usual activities which aid communication.

## F. Treatment of Adolescents

Although as noted by Warren, 'a new sub-speciality of adolescent psychiatry is developing in England and in the United States, with its own organisation' (The Association for the Psychiatric Study of Adolescents, England), most child psychiatrists assess and treat such adolescents as come their way.

Adolescents, unless they are immature early adolescents, are usually seen 'in their own right'. Which means that their appointments are not linked with parental appointments, except where a joint interview or a family meeting is planned. Parents may visit the social worker, or on occasion the psychiatrist at other times. With younger adolescents the form of treatment will depend on the stage reached by the patient. Many, in the free situation of the therapy room will make use of the opportunities for play and creativity sometimes with a remark, 'this is what my young brother would like to do' (playing with puppets) or 'I'll make a model for you' (playing cowboys and indians in the sand), or they may 'model' in clay, paint or build with construction sets. Regressive play may appear as therapy proceeds. Or talk may be interspersed with role playing or miming, or dressing up. Drawings or Winnicotts 'squiggles' often appeal to adolescents.

Older adolescents prefer 'just to talk' and in some cases their treatment is roughly similar to adult psychotherapy. Many, however, lack the motivation which this requires, they have come, at least initially, because of the concern of parents, or of society (perhaps from the courts).

If the adolescent can accept the psychiatrist in the role of adult confidant, and if the parents can accept this arrangement without interfering, the psychiatrist can give useful help; in other cases, where there is marked ambivalence to the psychiatrist testing-out and acting-out may occur. Missed appointments may indicate resistance or testing, but many adolescents find regular appointments do not suit their needs. In some clinics 'walk-in' appointments are available or clinics to which only adolescents come.

## G. Parental Aspects of the Child's Treatment

The mother's (or father's) part of therapy is usually taken on by the social worker and the practice and techniques of this skilled casework are more fully and appropriately described in books dealing with this subject than I could hope to do. Here we are dealing with aspects of the parent's treatment which impinge on the role of the psychiatrist who works closely with the social worker during the parallel treatment of the child and parent (Harrington,([12]) Hawkey and Barnes([13])). For the sake of convenience, and as this is still the more common practice, I will write as though the mother is attending.

Questions concerned with referral and the willingness of parents to trust the clinic sufficiently to accept treatment for their child lead on to considerations of on-going therapy. The importance of keeping the mother positively motivated towards the clinic, in order to secure continued treatment for the child, has been stressed by analysts (as Anna Freud puts it 'to prevent the child truanting from the analysis') but is, of course, also important for the sake of the mother and the whole family.

Parents often accept treatment because they see it as a way of removing symptoms and dealing with troublesome behaviour, and they turn deaf ears to explanations that treatment may change the child in other ways and that they will also have a part to play in treatment. The mother may have mixed feelings that the doctor (seen at least initially as the 'expert') is seeing the child, especially as she comes to realise that she is receiving therapy from another worker. She will already have had a conference with the psychiatrist in the early stages and may seek it again. It may be difficult to refuse the 'quick word' in the corridor but if the child is present it must be avoided. A request for a special appointment, unless indicated by the stage the therapy has reached with the agreement of the social worker, must also be refused.

In large clinics such difficulties may be averted by having one psychiatrist deal with the diagnostic evaluation and any follow-on needed with the parent(s), and another take over the therapy. However, it must be said that as well as the mother having an urge to talk to the psychiatrist who is treating her child the psychiatrist may have an unconscious wish to talk to the parent. This demonstrates a lack of confidence in his professional partner and will disrupt both the situation between the mother and the social worker and his treatment of the child. What is required is frequent reiteration of the team approach.

As well as being jealous of what the child is getting, the mother may find that what she is getting is difficult for her. A realisation that details of her own life and relationships, past and present, are relevant to what is happening to her child may make her feel exposed, and part of casework skill is to help her to feel able to reveal things in her own time through the confidence she feels in the clinic in general and in her social worker in particular.

Two factors are likely to prevent this happening. Where the mother has a relationship with the child which is abnormally close she may feel bereft if the child's behaviour changes, if he begins to look at her with new eyes, if his preoccupation seems to switch to the therapist. The need to continue her 'hot line' with the child may make her feel she cannot permit him to be close to anyone else, for fear that he will move away from her or reveal things about her. She may 'pump' the child on the way home, and eventually this will have the effect of censorship upon him, and he will come to feel as though his mother is really present with him during his therapeutic hour.

The other factor is the imbalance of family forces. A mother receiving individual casework may feel more threatened than when the whole family is involved, and may find it preferable to retain the predictable, disturbed behaviour of the patient than to face an alteration in behaviour which will change the balance within the family, and for which she may be blamed.

Another kind of balance is being sought by the therapists, between the need of the child for therapy and the needs of the mother herself, the need to keep the child attending at all costs and the need to deal honestly with both sides. Some analysts evade this problem by sending the child away for treatment and ignoring the parents, but this is not relevant to clinic practice.

Some mothers may be helped by being included in each stage of the child's treatment, though this has to be done without breaking the child's confidence. Some mothers are only too willing, at least at the beginning, that material they give the social worker should be used by the psychiatrist to speed the child's treatment, but may later resent this. In any case it may achieve little since the child may suspect that the things which come up in his sessions have been related by the mother, and he will be convinced that his secrets will be revealed to her.

The real answer is the 'therapeutic alliance' which develops for the mother as well as for the child. Interest shown in her for herself may be a new and rewarding experience for her, and her sessions with the social worker come to have a value for her irrespective of the child's treatment, and this brings a wish to continue for her own sake.

## H. Group Therapy in Child Guidance*

If group therapy is selected it must be as the method of choice, and as the best hope for the child. It is not to be thought of as a time saver, which it rarely is, since in many cases either the child or the mother needs to be seen individually as well as in the group.

*Parallel groups*

The arrangements are flexible, but commonly the children meet each week with the child psychiatrist or the psychotherapist, while at the same time the mothers meet with the social worker.

The group of mothers is likely to be rather different from the usual 'stranger' group carefully chosen to balance similarities and contrasts, so that no member becomes unduly dominant or is likely to antagonise the group. This can and does happen in a group of mothers who have come together because of the needs of their children. Some of the mothers are also likely to mingle during the week, and a certain amount of 'work' may be done (though without involving the whole group) especially as the children will also mix. The composition, size and activities of the mothers' group is not of paramount importance if the aim is discussion or behaviour modification, but if it is for a true group analytic approach, with the aim of the promotion of change through communication, experience, learning and insight then the usual protocol would be a balanced group of a size large enough not to be too depleted by the absence of one or two members, and the group requested not to meet between sessions. This may be difficult to achieve except in a large clinic, but it may be possible with a group of fathers (or mothers and fathers) who meet in the evenings, the children receiving individual treatment at other times (Durkin,[17] Slavson([18])).

*Children's Groups*

There are many ways in which children can be grouped, by age (emotional rather than chronological), by symptom (a group of encopretics or asthmatics), by diagnosis and need (neurotic or severely deprived).

The aim may be preventive, such as a group of preschool children, some at least of whom have experienced some deprivation, or it may aim at providing nurturant or 'primary' experiences, or at facilitating the working through of problems by play, creative activities or talk. The therapist may use comments and interpretations, or may be non-directive simply reflecting back what is happening.

*See Thompson,([14]) Walton([15]) and Bion.([16])

The group may consist of, for example, a number of 'latency' children with perhaps one or two younger children to facilitate regression and maturation, or a group of adolescents.

Peer grouping is usually appropriate for adolescents. The group may consist of early, middle or late adolescents, and may be of one or of both sexes. It is usually run on group analytic lines, sometimes with a co-therapist (Skynner,[19] Kraft[20])).

If the aim is socialisation, activities and projects may be introduced which may include co-operative ventures. Behaviour modification may also be practised in groups.

Anthony[21] describes three 'small' techniques for group treatment of kindergarten, latency and adolescent patients, using group-analytic techniques.

*(a). The 'small table' technique with kindergarten children (4–6 years)*

Anthony developed the idea of a round table with a central water trough, the remainder divided by removable barriers into a number of sections communicating by small access areas.

Each child has his own sector with his individual colour on his own set of toys. The therapist also has his own area and his own set of play equipment. In the early stages the children tend to play in their own territory in a parallel way, borrowing and interacting only with the therapist, later they encroach on or share one another's territory by scaling walls, burrowing underneath. They begin to borrow from each other, and still later the barriers may be removed and collective play themes, associations and phantasies develop.

The therapist remains largely passive, except in the initial stages, and he directs his interpretations towards the activity of the whole group of children.

*(b). The 'small room' technique with latency children*

After experimenting with various combinations of discussion plus activity groups, Anthony developed a technique designed to keep the children and therapist in close proximity to one another within a small space. The aim is towards group-analytic discussion but activity which develops spontaneously is not discouraged, but is then discussed. The small room is bare, except for a small table and some chairs. The six children and the therapist fill it, and Anthony stresses that they are all in the treatment situation together, there is no way out for any of them. At first the children feel uneasy and suspicious of the other children but more particularly of the therapist, who reflects everything that is happening back to them. As they begin to interact with one another and activity begins they continue to be aware of the therapist and of the comments he makes, as he interprets what is happening between the children and between the children and himself. Still later the children interpret what goes on between themselves.

Much depends on whether the children are girls or boys, and whether the therapist is of the same or the opposite sex.

Anthony finds this method particularly useful in acting out pre-delinquent children, and still uses for the less disturbed and more neurotic and anxious child the earlier model of discussion followed by activity.

## (c). The 'small circle' technique with adolescents

The room should be bare and scantily furnished, the circle slightly larger and the chairs more comfortable. The therapist interprets group activity and behaviour, and needs to be ready for the contracting and expanding of the group circle, which is part of a tendency of adolescent groups to regress and progress.

Questions of identity both individual and group, and adolescent crisis situations are to the forefront, and group themes phantasies and dreams are frequent. Anthony considers that mixed adolescent groups may be too inhibiting or too disturbing. (See also Frank,[22] and Ginott[23]).

## Bibliography and Further Reading

Items marked * are particularly important sources. Unnumbered references provide alternative sources to the reference quoted immediately above.

*1.  Isaacs, S. (1929) *The Nursery Years,* Routledge & Kegan Paul, London.
 2.  Lowenfeld, M. (1935) *Play in Childhood,* Victor Gollancz, London.
 3.  Klein, M. (1949) *The Psychoanalysis of Children,* Hogarth Press, London.
 4.  Klein, M. (1948) Infant analysis, in *Contributions to Psychoanalysis,* Hogarth Press, London.
 5.  Freud, A. (1928) *Introduction to the Technique of Child Analysis,* Nervous and Mental Disease Monograph Series, 48, New York.
 6.  Winnicott, D. W. (1971) *Playing and Reality,* Tavistock Publications, London.
 7.  Winnicott, D. W. (1971) *Therapeutic Consultations in Child Psychiatry,* Hogarth Press and the Institute of Psychoanalysis, London.
 8.  Winnicott, D. W. (1965) *The Maturational Processes and the Facilitating Environment,* Hogarth Press, London.
 9.  Burlingham, D. and Freud, A. (1944) *Infants without Families,* International Universities Press, New York.
*10. Dockar-Drysdale, B. (1968) *Therapy in child care,* Longmans, London.

11. Hickin, S. (1970/71) Group therapy with deprived children in a children's home, in *Groups, Annual Review of the Child Care Association,* **28,** 16.
12. Harrington, M. (1960) The integration of child therapy and casework, *J. Child Psychol. Psychiat.* **1,** 2, 113–120.
13. Hawkey, L., and Barnes, M. (1958) Collaboration within the therapeutic team, in *Ventures in Professional Cooperation* (ed. Barnes, M.)
*14. Thompson, S. and Kahn, J. H. (1970) *The Group Process as a Helping Technique,* Pergamon Press, Oxford.
*15. Walton, H. (1971) *Small Group Psychotherapy,* Penguin Books, Harmondsworth.
16. Bion, W. R. (ed.) (1961) *Experiences in Groups,* Tavistock Publications, London.
17. Durkin, H. E. (1954) *Group Therapy for Mothers of Disturbed Children,* Charles Thomas, Springfield, Illinois.
18. Slavson, S. R. (1958) *Child-centred Group Guidance of Parents,* International Universities Press, New York.
*19. Skynner, A. C. R. (1970/71) Group therapy with adolescent boys, in *Groups, Annual Review of the Child Care Association,* **18,** 16.
*20. Kraft, I. A. (1968) An overview of group therapy with adolescents, *Int. J. Grp. Psychother.* **18,** 4, 461–480.
*21. Anthony, E. J. (1957) Group-analytic psychotherapy with children and adolescents, in *Group Psychotherapy* (by Foulkes, S. H. and Anthony, E. J.) Penguin Books, Harmondsworth (revised edition 1973).
22. Frank, M. G. and Zilbach, J. (1968) Current trends in group therapy with children, *Int. J. Grp. Psychother.* **18,** 4, 447–460.
23. Ginott, H. (1961) *Group Psychotherapy with Children,* McGraw-Hill, London.

# CHAPTER 18

## *Termination*

We have been considering ways of keeping the treatment going for the child, but there does come a time when we have to begin to think of termination.

We have given a lot of attention to beginning, but ending is just as important as beginning. The reactions of the child to endings are instructive when, for example, therapist or child are ill or go on holiday. Sometimes the child can be prepared for these separations, sometimes they occur without warning. If the therapist leaves, the whole question of 'handing over' as opposed to termination needs' to be thrashed out, but neither should occur suddenly. Termination may occur suddenly if the parent just refuses to bring the child any more. Fortunately this is rare once treatment is well under way. The parent can usually be persuaded to bring the child for a final visit which the therapist can use to show that he is not rejecting the child, and also to prevent the damage which would result from the belief that parent and therapist are 'not friends'.

Treatment should not become a permanent crutch for the child (or parent) nor should the child be permitted a 'flight into illness' at the mere mention of termination in order to keep the treatment going. Therapists, too, need to examine closely any reactions they may have to some anxiety shown by the child as termination approaches, as they too may be motivated to continue. Allen([1]) has said 'treatment is started with the eventual goal of termination' and this goal should be kept in sight along the way.

Most therapists have tussled with the question of termination. Anna Freud([2]) takes the problem back to developmental stages, feeling that there may be no need to take the child further than most children are at his chronological age if development is going ahead satisfactorily, or we can ask whether the parents would have brought the child for treatment if his condition had been what it is today. This relies too heavily on symptomatic improvement. Successful treatment is seen as taking a step away from the untenable past and finding a better way of living.

We have to look at changes in the child's feelings and behaviour as shown during the therapeutic hour.

*Attitude to toys and play*

Is he less aggressive to the toys and less concerned about other children using them? Is there a change in his attitude to mess in the playroom (in either direction)? Is there a change in his attitude to time and other limits in his creative expressions and verbalisations? Is there less need to engage in regressive or aggressive play?

*Changes in feelings*

These are more important than behaviour. When the child first comes to treatment his emotions are diffuse and undifferentiated, his feelings often negative, and no longer attached to the people and situations which originally aroused them. Thus anger and hostility are at first non-specific, but later become sharpened and the child feels free to attach them where they belong, to brother or father or self. At the same time they are becoming less intense, as with the release of tension more positive feelings can emerge and he can move on to ambivalence. Thus he can care for, but occasionally spank, his baby brother (in the playroom and at home) instead of denying his negative feelings or projecting them. Similarly anxiety is at first diffuse and the child may be withdrawn, tense, garrulous or overanxious. Such a child is really immobilised, unable to think, to start (and certainly not to complete) anything. Fears possess him. Gradually the fears become more specific, relating to parents, siblings and others, are diluted by more positive attitudes and become milder and less pervasive. Gradually ambivalence gives way to a 'normal' separation of positive and negative attitudes which become attached to reality situations.

While all this is taking place the child needs a less and less intense and dependent relationship with the therapist.

We can see that when most, if not all, of this has been achieved the child himself is able to take a part in the termination of his treatment. Allen again: 'The end of treatment is affirming and reaffirming the differences the child perceives in himself, and the way in which old things have been used to provide structure for the new.'

Therapy has been an important experience for the child and this should be in no way denied, so it is important for him to see that the experience is not lost, that although therapy will have its own ending and become another past, the new qualities which have come into being will last when it is over.

The child needs time to live through the emotions aroused by this new separation. He may openly show anxiety and should be helped to express this, but it should not ordinarily be seen as a reason to continue. Finally it is up to the child to decide how he ends, jauntily, regretfully, aggressively or in a casual, friendly manner (see Axline[3]).

Termination for child and parent can be seen as interdependent, but to a degree it is also independent. Usually, since the therapists consult together frequently a plan for simultaneous termination may be made; the child and parent began together, they finish together. If a follow-up interview is planned this too may be kept together, although in some cases the parent alone may keep it. In other cases the parent may continue when the child finishes. The parent may have been slow to respond to the opportunity for her own needs, and is therefore a step or two behind the child. She must not be left in mid-air, if her problems are more serious, or her personality more fragile than was thought at first. When termination approaches the parent as well as the child may feel anxiety, but this is not necessarily a reason for continuing visits to the clinic.

## Bibliography and Further Reading

Item marked * is a particularly important source.

*1.  Allen, F. (1942) *Psychotherapy with Children,* Norton, New York.
 2.  Freud, A. (1965) *Normality and Pathology in Childhood,* Hogarth Press, London.
     Axline, V. (1964) *Dibs: In Search of Self,* Penguin Books, Harmondsworth.

## CHAPTER 19

# Treatment of Individual Children

## A. James's Treatment

This was carried out over 14 months and was mainly non-directive, though occasional comments and interpretations were made. Sessions were weekly, later fortnightly and the last two at monthly intervals. During the treatment James's father remarried, and his school was changed. The account is necessarily much abbreviated.

The first interview with the psychiatrist indicated the characteristic way in which this intelligent but extremely anxious 7-year-old met a challenge by bringing his feelings out into the open rather than by silence and withdrawal.

### First part

For the first few weeks James continued to wonder what the clinic could mean for him, about limits (especially time), about sharing, but particularly about his relationship with me.

He talked fast, often jumping from one topic to another and jumping around himself, but he never mentioned his family. He could not play, though sometimes he banged the sand about or flung some onto the floor. One day he suddenly threw some sand at me and threatened to shoot me with the dart gun. 'You are feeling angry?' I said. 'Why can't I stay with you, why do I have to go, ever?' I told him that this did not mean that I did not care about him. From this point he began to communicate; first of his feelings about school, 'that hard work', contrasting it with the play school his brother goes to; of his strict teacher, and the housekeeper who 'won't let me play out after tea, ever'. He feels he can't get near her. About the girls who looked after him, especially 'long-legged Jean' who left to get married. 'I loved her.' He looked at my long legs. 'Are you married?' he wanted to know. I asked him how he would like it to be. 'I know you're married really, your wedding ring,' pause, 'But you'll be here. Jean went away.' He told me about an older woman who came. 'She stole Daddy's drink. Daddy shouldn't have to be worried, he's so busy.' (The housekeeper has said this to James.)

*Central part*

After about nine weekly sessions James suddenly began to use clay. He slapped it around saying it was 'to practise for school' (they do not have clay at his school). He found a discarded clay figure in the waste bucket and began to paint it black. 'Black?' I said. 'Black' said James, 'Coal black, inky black, night black,' then, shouting, 'Dead black.' He looked pale, began to tremble, came and stood close to me. Neither of us spoke. Then he gave me the figure, 'to keep till next time'.

On the next visit he began to speak of his mother, and of the many photographs of her in his house. Of one he said 'It's not black, it's her wedding dress. The one I like best. White.' He began to dance about laughing, acting the clown. 'I don't think you're feeling happy', I told him. He gave me a sad abstracted look, then went to the sand, making a big castle. 'No-one can get out' he said. I nodded (he and I are stuck in the therapy). He picked up a naked doll and painted the body black, the legs in bright yellow and red stripes (the sadness and the denial), looking at me and shaking his head sadly. He turned away and busied himself making some 'milk' with white paint in a little cup. He offered it to me. 'You want me to drink it?' I asked. He snatched it away, 'It might make you ill'. 'My mother was ill', he explained. 'She went to hospital, we thought we could cope', pause, 'One night she got in a muddle with her tablets and took too many. At least I think that's what happened. She didn't know what she was doing.' I asked about the milk he'd made. 'She could have been poisoned, someone might have given her some milk that wasn't good, perhaps by mistake. My mother didn't mean to die', fiercely. 'She didn't mean to die', I repeated. 'To leave me', he said. Memories and phantasies came flooding, 'In the morning I couldn't wake her up. She went off in an ambulance and Auntie Joan from next door came in and dressed me. Rupert was asleep. Later I asked my father "Is she dead?"; he said "No". I wondered about it.' 'You wondered. "Could she really be dead? My mother in the white dress." 'Now let's play.' He finished the session with active play with me.

Next time he played the whole while in the soft sand in a lively and aggressive fashion with cowboys and indians, wanting me to join in. When I warned him that time would be up in 5 minutes, he quickly buried all the figures in the sand, 'So the next boy won't find them'. He asked for confirmation of next week's appointment.

Next time he brought a tooth which had come out, he gave it to me. 'I love playing now' he said.

Next time he told me he was going on holiday, to Spain. 'Rupert is going too, I'll be brown when I get back and I'll come straight to see you.'

At this stage father reported that James was doing better at school. He was arranging for him to have some coaching at home. During the holiday he met the woman he later married.

James seemed moody and tentative on his return. He had brought Rupert up to my room saying, 'He wants to play', but was so aggressive towards him that Rupert soon left. I commented that he had found it more difficult to share the toys and me than he had expected. He said in a surly voice that he didn't know if he'd be coming any more, 'I have a teacher in the house now,' 'You think I am a teacher?' I asked. 'Well, I see you to help me learn. Bringing Rupert was Daddy's idea too' he said. 'You seem upset', I commented. A tear ran down his cheeks, 'I can't seem to play today' he said.

Next time he wanted to talk about 'people's bodies'. He'd 'peeped' and seen the girl next door sitting on the lavatory. He'd climbed into bed with Grandma, 'I wanted to feel her chest', but Grandma was cross. He asked Daddy what ladies are like without their clothes and Daddy was cross. He told me 'We have a lady coming to see us. Daddy met her on holiday', then went off to find some girl's 'frilly pants' to wash. He went back to talking about other children coming to the clinic, and wanting to daub their wall paintings; he also behaved regressively in a way he had not done before, sucking the baby's bottle, and sucking his thumb. He told me he had asked Daddy to dress him, 'but he wouldn't'. 'Sometimes it's easier if you're little' I ventured. 'She likes Rupert', he said.

Next time there was more about 'the lady. She's thin and doesn't eat dinners or teas. Will she stay alive?' He began to play in the sand, burying all the soldiers, then left some lying on top. 'My grandfather put unburied soldiers in their graves', he said. 'You seem interested in graves.' 'I never saw my mother's, you know' he said. Then 'Daddy has taken down all her photos.' 'All?' I queried, 'Even the wedding one' he said. 'Perhaps you are thinking about Daddy getting married.' 'One of them has to be dead', he said. He looked straight at me. 'I thought perhaps you could die, but I was frightened. I didn't want you to die' (I knew he was referring to the milk). 'It wasn't really poison, only paint and water' he said, 'I thought I might get my mummy back, you couldn't really be my mummy.' 'But now you are going to have a real mummy', I said.

Next time he told me the date of the marriage, 'It's great, we haven't had a mummy for a long time', then expressed concern that she'll like Rupert better than him. Rupert has started at James's school now, 'Everyone likes him', he said. 'Everyone?' 'Except you perhaps.' This was said with a grin, and I didn't really have to remind him, 'But you said I couldn't be your mummy'.

On the last visit before the wedding he told me 'Daddy took me to see my mother's grave. I asked him. We took that dead mummy some flowers.' He told me about the clothes he'll be wearing at the wedding.

*After the wedding, Moving towards termination*

Stepmother is a smart level-headed young woman who sees things clearly and seeks a practical solution. She firms father up to tackle his mother and James's school is changed to a more permissive one where he can receive remedial help. She accepts that James's emotional needs are at the Oedipal stage. He has been trying to observe her in the nude and has shown interest in the marital bed. She is quite tolerant and amused, though father is not. She has found some flaws in Rupert, and she accepts James at the stage he has reached. It is clear that she will not reject him. It is also clear that she and father feel that the family has all it needs and that unless there is a crisis we must work towards termination.

During this time, James at first showed some upset which soon passed. After the wedding he seemed strained, told me 'We're moving. To London I think. I may not be able to give you my address.' He banged about angrily in the sand. It seemed he thought he would not be seeing me any more. Next time he told me they were only moving to the next street, and told me that he was now going to a new school. 'My special teacher knows you. Rupert can stay at that old work school.' He began to play with the doll's house, putting mother and father in a big bed, then added a boy remarking 'I don't go in their bed'. He took the boy out and put a baby in (himself or the baby he thought stepmother might have). He talked about things at home. 'She might really be my mummy', but then took the mother figure and put it through the rollers of the mangle. 'I'm not sure' he said. Next time he was quoting the remedial teacher, 'I'm really artistic, I made up a poem and Miss S. wrote it down', and stepmother 'We played draughts and I didn't mind losing, I used to you know.' He looked straight at me. 'I didn't call her mummy at first. I wasn't sure. But now I do.'

He played again with the soldiers in the sand, he seemed to be wondering whether to bury them. 'It was true about grandfather you know.' 'About burying soldiers? Yes, I know it was true' (grandfather worked for War

Graves). 'It was all true, but a long time ago,' said James. I remarked that we wouldn't have many more times together. 'I know. It isn't so bad with Rupert now,' he said 'Now that I'm getting clever at school.'

On the last visit James was in a hurry. Mummy was going with him to a concert at his school. 'It's a play really. I have a part. I've learnt it all. Daddy can't go but it doesn't matter. Rupert will be in bed.' He arranged the dolls' house with mother, father and two boys sitting round the table. 'I'll shut the door now' he said. He left his coat behind, and as he ran off with it he called, 'You could come to the concert, too, except that there mightn't be a ticket.'

## B. Heather, aged 9 (see p. 72)

*Heather's treatment*

Heather used the small round playroom to make a little home. She arranged the small tables and used boxes for seats, the dolls' cots were beds, with paper for sheets and balsa blocks for pillows, a small chest of drawers became the cooker. She sewed together scraps of material to make curtains for the tiny windows; when Christmas came she made paper chains. Within this home Heather played out the themes of her life, her babyhood, her toddler years with her happy, then ailing, then dying mother, her mother's death. Sometimes she was the mother, sometimes the child, or I played some of the parts, or she used dolls; over and over as though she would never move on. One day she brought a photograph of her mother which no one knew she had, and the next time a minute doll which her grandmother had given her, 'Grannie called it a dinky doo', she said and for the first time she smiled. Now she introduced other characters into her play, her father, her teenage sister, her grandmother, her teachers and the girls at school. At school they reported that she was talking and skipping with the girls at school, she smiled at the headmaster when she took him his cup of tea in the morning. She began to cook meals for her father and sister. They went for a seaside holiday together. Father's comment, 'Heather's getting quite pretty'.

## C. Stephen, aged 5 (see p. 127)

*Stephen's treatment*

Stephen did not speak for his first six sessions in the playroom. He stood, a sturdy little figure just inside the door, not moving, with his eyes fixed on the dolls' house. I moved it onto the floor and got down myself. Stephen sat crosslegged beside me, his arms folded. I began to move some of the dolls and furniture about saying nothing. There were some cars in the garage, Stephen reached out and pulled one of them towards him. He played with the cars, keeping them very close to the house, they were coming and going as though they were people. At the second session I began a running commentary about who the cars seemed to be and what they were doing. Stephen shook his head if I made a mistake. The mother car did not go far away and never without the children, who seemed to be very well behaved. They went to school and to church. The daddy car went to work, and sometimes went out with a friend. The mummy car went shopping and came home again. 'Nothing much seems to happen in this family', I said. Stephen pushed one of the cars and brought out a little red mail van. He made it clear that this van was himself. The red mail van was very naughty. He banged about a lot and bumped into the other children cars. The mummy car kept sending him to the garage, but he kept getting out. He kept needing to be filled up with petrol but sometimes it came out again and he couldn't have any more.

As time went on the family would go farther and farther from the house and have picnics and all sorts of exciting adventures.

Stephen began to use the dolls' house figures and to talk. Now there were two Stephens, a boy in a red blazer was the good Stephen and the little red mail van was the naughty Stephen. The good Stephen went into the house and sat on the lavatory but the bad Stephen went into the garage and squirted petrol all over the floor. Stephen laughed a lot about that. (His mother reported that the soiling had cleared up and that she and Stephen were having 'great fun'.) Soon after this day the little red mail van went too fast along a bumpy road and fell down a hole, 'And that's the end of him' said Stephen.

These two short cases indicate the use of Child Psychiatry in organically based conditions.

*Fiona* was a 14-year-old girl suffering from Turner's syndrome (chromosome abnormality). She was dwarfed with a webbed neck so that her disproportionally large head appeared to sit straight on her shoulders. She was plump and squat, but secondary female sex (breasts, pubic hair) characteristics had not developed and menstruation was absent. In her case, however, there was no intellectual retardation and, in spite of her grotesque appearance, she was of average intelligence.

Those dealing with Fiona were aware that there was not going to be any change for the better in her condition, and each in his own way tried to help her. Her parents indulged her at the expense of her younger normal sibling.

Her mother, herself a very pretty woman, bought Fiona attractive 'teenage' clothes, but Fiona would never try them on in shops nor look at herself in the mirror. The Headmistress of the secondary modern school put her in the A stream where she could not cope with the work but where the other children were less likely to make fun of her. The various local organisations, Guides, St. John's Ambulance Cadets and Church Groups, fell over backwards to fill all her leisure moments. Mother was always trying to make special arrangements for her, such as getting her music lessons (she had no aptitude) or a 'little job' (she was under age), and constantly urged the family doctor and the paediatrician to 'do something'. The doctor saw Fiona every week, but, at a loss how to behave, set up a joking relationship with her, calling her 'freak' and kidding that she would have to be 'put down'; the paediatrician, egged on by mother, wondered whether Fiona would feel more 'normal' if she achieved a menstrual period and referred her to a gynaecologist.

Fiona was brought to the notice of the child psychiatrist as she was gradually withdrawing from all her activities, first her evening gatherings, and then refusing to go to school. She was said to be depressed and irritable.

At a case conference held at the doctor's surgery it was clear that none of the participants had been able to face up to their feelings about Fiona's condition, and there was denial of her feelings all round. Fiona and her mother, when seen in joint interview, presented smiling faces. Mother, speaking brightly, answered for Fiona. When seen alone Fiona was feeling that people arranged things for her as if she were not there, and talked about her as though she did not understand. She knew they wanted to give her a period so she would be like other girls, but 'I know I can't have babies', she said. She felt that she had no choice between keeping up appearances totally, smiling and carrying on with everything, or giving in completely, and hiding her head. She was relieved to be able to take off her mask and reveal a very deep and realistic sorrow. Mother, too, found some solace in being able to ventilate her anger and sadness about her daughter's condition, and to accept that the hostile feelings she sometimes had towards her were normal. Mother and Fiona — indeed the whole family — were able to achieve a much more workable way of living together. Fiona began to feel a real person albeit an unusual one. One indication was that mother now chose clothes which played down rather than dramatised Fiona's anatomical peculiarities. Fiona began to find her own interests and talents and to decide herself what she would and would not do.

*Alistair,* aged 9, the eldest and only boy in a two-child family was referred for restless, cheeky and disruptive behaviour and poor progress at school in spite of apparently good ability; at home he was awkward and defiant. His younger sibling was already catching him up academically.

The history revealed that mother had haemorrhages and toxaemia during pregnancy. Alistair was jaundiced and was in an incubator for 2 days. He was an irritable, crying baby, who had problems with feeding and, later, speech. He was whining and clinging and always wanted mother to do things for him she thought he should do himself, like tying his shoelaces or doing up buttons. Father thought this was because he was clumsy: he pointed out to mother that Alistair dropped things and was poor at catching or kicking a ball, but mother was irritated with him.

On examination, Alistair was cross-lateral, his co-ordination was poor and he was clumsy at manipulation. There were minor neurological abnormalities. His speech was immature.

Psychological tests showed a discrepancy of 25 points between his Verbal IQ (114) and his Performance IQ (89). He had a high error score on the Bender Gestalt and the record was immature. There were visuo-motor difficulties. An electroencephalogram suggested that there was a minor degree of brain damage. These findings were useful, in that the parents and the school could see that Alistair had real difficulties in learning. An accurate assessment of his needs was made, and remedial help was arranged as well as guidance for his teacher. The temperature was cooled generally and mother was able to respond to Alistair in a much warmer way, while father's sympathy was able to take a practical form in helping Alistair with the skills he did have.

### PART V

# Family Therapy

*Historically the emphasis initially placed on the disturbed child, has shifted to the mother and child then to both parents and child and finally to the whole family, and to the community (Prince,([1]) Martin and Knight,([2]) Broadley,([3]) Brown and Rutter,([4]) Beels and Ferber,([5]) McGregor([6])).*

*Ackerman([7]) has pointed out that the change was long overdue, that concentration on the pathology of the child meant that 'the tail was wagging the dog', and he has stressed 'the interlocking pathology of the family, extending over three generations'.*

*Just as child therapy is different from adult therapy and groups of parents different from groups of 'strangers', so family therapy is different from both individual and group therapy. The family is a 'natural' group, which existed before therapy began and will continue when it ends; it also functions outside the treatment sessions. The family group has come from previous families and generations and future families and generations will stem from it.*

---

## CHAPTER 20

## Basis for Family Therapy

The family meets and gratifies many fundamental needs of parents and children, but these needs may be warped or pathological, and the result may be unhealthy and collusive behaviour arising from the interlocking vulnerabilities of the family. Questions of family functioning and dynamics were dealt with in Chapter 4, and it may be useful to re-read that section before proceeding.

Variations in the practice of family therapy depend on the orientation of the therapist or school of therapy, and an impression of a variety of approaches will be given, but broadly family therapy may be seen as an approach (mainly dynamic) orientated towards the family as a whole, during which the 'problem' is re-enacted in the here and now situation, and during which the family functioning and the rules by which the family operates are demonstrated.

## A. Advantages of Family Therapy

### 1. Location of the problem

It is claimed that family therapy puts the problem back where it belongs, in the family where it has arisen and where the genesis and continuance of the symptoms of the identified patient has happened.

### 2. Time factors

(a) Family intervention is more likely than individual therapy to prevent the child's condition from becoming chronic. The 'symptom' may have originated as a cry for help and a need to bring changes in the family group, but if this fails and the crisis is not resolved for the child, the symptom is perpetuated and incorporated into family patterns of reaction. Thus the role the child is playing loses its aim, the whole family situation becomes fossilised, and long-term treatment is required.

(b) The child is with his family or with individual members of it far more than with anyone else. Howells,[8] taking the span of the first 10 years of life has estimated that the child spends the greatest amount of time sleeping (29·7 percent of 24 hours) but almost as much time with his mother (23·45 percent) siblings (18·62 percent) father (12·72 percent) and more with adult relatives (4·79 percent) than with peers and teachers at school (4·27 percent). The inclusion of the preschool years affects the latter figures, but on the other hand at home he is often in a one-to-one relationship with his mother, whereas at school he usually has to share his teacher with thirty other children.

(c) Interaction within the family continues outside the therapy and hopefully in a more healthy way. The family also does 'homework' following sessions, so that a good deal of 'work' is done between sessions resulting in at best progress, at worst regression, but at least change.

(d) Skynner([9]) in particular claims that because family motivations and ability to respond and contribute to this kind of therapy appear quickly, it is possible to estimate possible progress after two or three meetings, and a decision taken at this time as to whether it is economic to continue, or whether some other approach would be more suitable to this family.

### 3. Need to involve both parents (Hallowitz([10]))

Centrally placed are the parents. Satir([11]) has called them 'the architects of the family', and considers that since marital aspects greatly affect parenting these must be tackled if the child is to be helped. The father may not see it as part of his role to 'trail along to clinics', considering this to be 'women's work', but if from the outset it is made clear that his presence is required as 'head of the family', and that no-one else can speak for him he is usually ready to take part. The whole business of family therapy often makes sense to him more quickly than it does to the mother.

### 4. Need to involve siblings (see Ackerman, p. 62)

(a) The siblings may be equally disturbed although in a different, and perhaps less obtrusive way, e.g. withdrawn rather than 'acting out'.

(b) The siblings may differ markedly from the picture given of them by the parents.

(c) The parents often behave quite differently to the 'normal' siblings than to the 'patient'; with the former they show warmth and flexibility and awareness of needs, with the latter there is constriction and turning away.

(d) The siblings react differently to the 'patient' than they do to one another. In one session Susie, aged 3, said to her mother regarding the scapegoated Brian, 8, 'We don't like Brian, do we?'

(e) During therapy, in a situation where the 'patient' is too inhibited or discouraged to speak, a sibling may by making vital contributions speed the therapy along, and in a way which may be more acceptable to the parents.

## 5. Need of the child for the family when the family is unable to meet the need

Ackerman([12,13]) has pointed to the social alienation and disharmony in individuals' relationship with society and with one another today, and May has diagnosed the current malaise as aloneness, anxiety and emptiness. This leads to a sense of lostness and aloneness, especially in adolescence. Although it is said that the family is breaking apart, many young people do turn to their families in distress from failure, to find a safe place in the world and to reassure them of their loveableness and value. Satir has said that children need their parents to 'validate' them but many parents, deprived or with problems of their own, are unable to do this or to give the reassurance. They need so much themselves that they have little to spare for the children. The 'patient' (some weakness in the child, resemblance to a despised relative, circumstances at the time of the birth) seems to be the 'last straw' and a threat to the uneasy stability of the family. Family therapy brings this out into the open and helps the members to make more realistic adjustments to each other.

## 6. Strengths and growth potential in the family (Ackerman, p. 61)

The family has a potential for growth and realignment of forces. Different members will move at different paces during family treatment, but this gives elasticity and allows vulnerable members time to manoeuvre and develop at their own pace.

## 7. Use in 'poor prognosis' families

Family therapy may be successful where other methods are likely to fail. Certain families may find the 'whole family' approach more relevant especially if meetings are less frequent, especially 'low esteem' families (Minuchin and Montalvo([14,15])).

## 8. Diagnosis

The family dynamics are seen in action. This cannot be reproduced in any other way.

## B. Disadvantages

### 1. Diagnosis, lack of a proper diagnostic procedure

Some critics consider that although a 'family diagnosis' is made there is no diagnosis for the 'patient'. Howells, for example, follows the usual diagnostic procedure at his intake interviews, but others may not do so, and there is a fear that some pathological condition in the 'patient' may be missed.

### 2. Forcing an ideal or stereotype on the family

Some ideal or stereotype of what family life and family communication should be, whether of models worked out by 'experts', the social 'norm' or from the therapist's own childhood, is imposed on the family. This may be done overtly as in the behaviour modelling techniques, or covertly by the attitude of the therapist. This is particularly liable to happen with low esteem or inadequate families, who may already have attempted to adopt such a stereotype (from outside models) which may be quite inappropriate for the family or for the individuals in it. This takes away from the dignity which the family may have.

### 3. Excessive emphasis on family pathology, ignoring strengths

This follows on from the above. It ignores the fact that health can be achieved in different ways in different families, and that situations where they have coped well in the past must be valued and may give clues about future help.

### 4. Reinforcement of family pathology

However, and this is most important, the family may block or reinforce one another in faulty methods of coping which become more entrenched, or take refuge in collective defences and denials.

### 5. Exposure of therapist

This really presupposes a weakness in the therapist. As we shall see, he is more in the thick of things in family therapy, is liable to be attacked by the family, and any idiosyncrasies he may have about family life are laid bare.

Also the violent interactions which may take place during a session may alarm a therapist into sidestepping important issues.

## C. Special Characteristics of Family Group Therapy

Family therapists note that they tend to be more free, spontaneous and active than in 'stranger' group therapy, and explanations have been sought for this. There are great differences in the strengths of the family members, from maturity, role and assumption. In the children (and also in some families the adults), self-control is limited. The family group is ideally placed because of its common psychopathology to collude in blocking vital communication. This calls for a more active and controlling role from the therapist.

However, the opposite aspect, i.e. that the family does hold the 'key', and that however knowledgeable the therapist may be he does not know as much about the family as they do themselves, enables the therapist to avoid the 'expert' role and take part openly in the interaction with the family, knowing that there is no possibility of his remarks being passed on incorrectly or out of context.

It has also been suggested that the therapist reacts intuitively to keep himself a real figure in order to prevent projections on to him from the family, and to keep transference reactions within the family. This is certainly the result, and the fact that primitive transferences already operating within the family are kept there is one of the reasons why such rapid changes are possible in family therapy. Further results of the greater activity of the therapist are that there is less regression among family members, and that it lessens the danger of fixing family pathology.

The kind and degree of activity varies, depending on the orientation of the therapist, and the kind of families they select for treatment. Variations include beginning in a more structured way, and then letting the family take over, or keeping the structure throughout; letting the family start with minimal interventions throughout, or with the therapist becoming more active as therapy proceeds and so on. Interventions tend to be more frequent than interpretations, for the families make the interpretations themselves.

## D. Selection of Cases for Family Therapy

Most family therapists, as they extend their experience and their expertise, find that more families are suitable for this form of therapy than they thought at first. Are there some families who may not be suitable?

Some families decide themselves that they are not suitable, or that they cannot cope with this kind of therapy.

Skynner[16] concludes that two other kinds are unsuitable, at least initially. Firstly families where the parents are very immature, the mother perhaps still in the dependency phase of infancy. Such a mother might receive individual therapy while the rest of the family attends group sessions, which the mother eventually joins. A similar procedure might be followed where one parent (or both) has severe neurotic problems (but with the beginning integration of personality which makes the procedure possible). Here parallel treatment for parent and child would be preferred initially, but later the whole family might be involved together.

Ackerman[12] excludes similar families, i.e. those on the verge of disintegration and those where there is long-standing psychic conflict in one or more members.

Most other families are suitable for some form of family therapy. Skynner[16] treats a wide variety, but finds the family approach particularly useful where the scapegoat, wonder boy or sick person may be considered the patient (though not necessarily the referred one).

Ackerman[13] considers family therapy to be particularly useful where the 'victim' is trapped within the family situation and cannot escape to the outside, while Satir[11] finds it useful in families of low esteem but also in crisis situations, in employment, marriage, delinquency, adolescence, etc. Howells, with his wide-ranging approach, welcomes every kind of family.

## Bibliography and Further Reading

Items marked * are particularly important sources. Unnumbered references provide alternative sources to the reference quoted immediately above.

1. Prince, G. S. (1961) A clinical approach to parent-child interaction, *J. Child Psychol. Psychiat.* **2**, 3, 169–184.
2. Martin, F. and Knight, J. (1962) Joint interviews as part of intake procedure in a child psychiatric clinic, *J. Child Psychol. Psychiat.* **3**, 1, 17–26.
3. Broadley, L. P. (1967) *Expanding Theory and Practice in Family Therapy*, Family Service Association, New York.
4. Brown G. and Rutter, M. (1966) The measurement of family activities and relationships, *Human Relations* **19**, 3, 241–263.
*5. Beels, C. C. and Ferber, A. (1969) Family Therapy: a view, *Family Process* **8**, 2, 280–318.
6. MacGregor, R. (1970) Group and family therapy: Moving into the present and letting go of the past, *Int. J. Grp. Psychother.* **20**, 4, 495–515.

7. Ackerman, N. *et al.* (1970) Childhood disorders and interlocking pathology in family relationships, in *The Child in his Family.* (eds. Anthony, E. J. and Koupernik, C.), Wiley-Interscience, New York.

8. Howells, J. G. (1972) Ipswich 1000 family survey, in *Family Therapy for Child Psychiatrists* (ed. Howells, J. G.), S. C. P. Reports.

*9. Skynner, A. C. R. (1969) A group-analytic approach to conjoint family therapy, *J. Child Psychol. Psychiat.* **10**, 2, 81–106.

10. Hallowitz, D. *et al.* (1957) The treatment process with both parents together, *Am. J. Orthopsychiat.* **27**, 3, 587–601.

11. Satir, V. (1967) *Conjoint Family Therapy,* Science and Behaviour Books, Palo Alto.

*12. Ackerman, N. (1966) *Treating the Troubled Family,* Basic Books, New York.
Ackerman, N. (1958) *Psychodynamics of Family Life,* Basic Books, New York.

13. Ackerman, N. (1958) Toward an integrative therapy of the family, *Am. J. Psychiat.* **114**, 727–733.

14. Minuchin, S. and Montalvo, B. (1967) Techniques for working with disorganized low socio-economic families, *Am. J. Orthopsychiat.* **37**, 4, 880–887.

15. Minuchin, S. *et al.* (1967) *Families of the Slums,* Basic Books, New York.

16. Skynner, A. C. R. (1967) Indications and contraindications for conjoint family therapy, *Br. J. soc. Psychiat.* **15**, 248.

## CHAPTER 21

# Family Therapy in Action

## A. Schools of Family Therapy

These vary from group-analytic type therapies to behaviour modelling therapies; to give a representative sample I have chosen Ackerman, Skynner, Satir, Lieberman and Howells. (Again, with apologies, for the brief accounts cannot do justice to the richness of their work.)

### Skynner

Skynner's([1,2]) method is based on group analytic therapy, with the aim of helping the family to work out its transference distortions and failures of communication with themselves and with the therapist. He stresses the importance of looking for what is missing, i.e. what is 'concealed and denied and so not communicated'. He does this by throwing the problem back to the family and by reflecting back to them what they present to him in terms of non-communication or of needs of family members which are not being met.

He affirms the authority and knowledge which the family have, which is greater than that of the therapist who is included in the treatment process because of his expertise in communication; thus he sees himself as facilitating the work done by the family.

In therapy all communications arise spontaneously from the family, and all family members are expected to take part. Non-verbal are given equal importance with verbal communications. The therapist involves himself in the family's difficulties and tries to understand why the family is seeking help at this time. He does not take or have a history available so that he is involved from the start in what is happening. 'A detailed history enables the therapist to understand only intellectually and in advance, out of time with the true rhythm of the family and out of touch with its living experience.' He asks the family about the 'symptom', what it is trying to say, what effect it has on other members of the family and for an account of family interactions

209

centring round the symptom. This brings the actual conflict situation into the therapy situation and most families are able to carry on from there. Apart from these initial questions activity is reserved for occasions when communication is being restricted, and to preserve his function of representing the demands of reality. He criticises Ackerman for 'excessive activity'; his own activity seems to vary somewhat. He does sometimes, as he admits himself 'take sides' but considers that this involves him more fully in the treatment process, and when treating less intelligent and less sophisticated families he focuses on behaviour modelling, and by his spontaneous behaviour helps the family to behave more freely.

Practical details are: families attend for three-weekly sessions of 1½ hours, all members of the family attend, arrangements are informal the family and therapist sitting in a circle with play materials in the centre. (The children however are invited to take a seat and participate verbally.) If one member does not attend (he may be the most disturbed member or he may have been elected to keep the family's problem at home) the family are invited to talk about this member, and it may in fact turn out that the therapist is being cast in his role. If one parent does not attend it may be because he (she) is unable to share the children with the partner in therapy until they have had their needs met.

Assessment of progress is made after about three sessions and some families may drop out at this stage, but usually not more than ten sessions in all are needed.

*Ackerman*

Ackerman[3,4] also stresses the authority of the family and sees the therapist both as conductor and as enabler who helps the family to bring its restitutory powers to bear on the situation. He starts off knowing more about the family than Skynner seeks to know, and commencing with the presenting problem he asks the family what it has to say about family relationships in general and impaired functioning in particular. He takes into account any immediate stresses within or outside the family. As these become clarified he seeks to cut across the established rules of play in the family, forcing the members to be more open with each other. He seeks both the reorganisation of the conscious facets of personality which have been integrated into family roles, and also some change in the unconscious facets. Parallel to this goes his role as a guide and educator.

*Satir*

Satir([5]) worked originally with the Palo Alto group with their special interest in schizophrenia and double-bind phenomena and she sees the basic need in 'troubled families' as a need for improved (more open and honest) communication, and greater confidence of the family members (particularly the marital pair) in themselves.

Her therapy is by model role modification, considering that the parents have received inadequate models from their parents (sex and mastery) and that the children in their turn have received inadequate models from them. She also clarifies roles and gets the family to see 'who is what and to whom'.

She sees the therapist as a model and teacher, who must also be a real person to the family, sharing to a degree their way of verbalising, making jokes, using colloquialisms etc.

She conducts firmly throughout. Her first aim is to reduce anxiety, and she starts with the marital pair, not in the present (which might be too threatening) but in the past, making a 'family chronology'. She helps the family to see that they are not as bád as they think they are, that they are functionally, rather than actually, helpless. She brings in the 'patient' and other children, but if these are very young they would not be invited to every session. Each attending member is fully involved, and no member is allowed to act out or block communication completely. No-one is allowed to speak for anyone else, but the need to keep everyone involved is kept to the forefront.

Current communication and its survival content is analysed. Satir clarifies and explains what is going on in simple terms over and over again, and brings it back each time to the whole family.

The treatment is not open ended, a plan is usually made for six sessions (of 1 or 1½ hours), then the situation is reassessed, but Satir is very flexible in her approach and uses many special variations.

She has said that her methods are most appropriate to disorganised and unsophisticated families, and indeed they seem particularly suited to them, in that she abandons distance, uses the means of communication to which they are accustomed, and joins the affective life of the family, experiencing the intensity of feeling within the family as though she were a family member. At the same time she demonstrates new ways of communicating and behaving to them.

*Learning theory techniques in family therapy*

Greater interest in these techniques in the sphere of family therapy has come about in a number of ways, first from the breaking down of barriers between the schools of therapy, second because of the greater activity of the therapist, and parallel with this the increased interest in non-verbal communication in family therapy.

Observation of family interaction is clearer if behaviour rather than feeling is picked up, and stimulus-response relationships pinpointed. By concentrating on observable responses, particularly sequences of behaviour which occur frequently, the therapist may be able to see vital clues that trigger off those sequences, and this may form a basis for direct intervention (this is useful in marital therapy also).

Mr and Mrs Jones (p. 155) had become bogged down in a stimulus-response vicious circle, whereby the sight of Mrs J. with her head in a book and/or the sight of the piled-up unwashed dishes in the sink caused her husband to go off to the pub on his own, where he would make some plan so that she would be unable to go out to work. Sometimes at the weekend he would start taking his car engine to pieces, 'even bringing it into the kitchen' said Mrs Jones, adding 'I hate that car', instead of taking the family out; thus punishing the children as well. The end result would be that she would snatch up a book 'to escape' her violent thoughts against him, and the scratchiness of the children.

When the therapist, instead of listening to the separate recitals of what had happened, pointed to the trigger mechanism and to its repetitiveness, and asked the couple to note the number of times the cycle had occurred between meetings and later to note occasions when there had been a different outcome, there was a change both in behaviour and relationships which had not been apparent in weeks of purely verbal interaction.

It is claimed that an additional advantage is that observation rather than insight may allow more accurate intervention. Moreover such observable data can be quantified and provide a measure of objective change which can be utilised in therapy.

*Modelling, role-playing empathy*

It has been noted that the therapist is more active in family therapy, and techniques such as modelling age, gender, or role-appropriate behaviour to members of the family comes naturally to the more active or, as they are sometimes called, 'transparent' family therapists. This may take the form of demonstrating through his own behaviour how to give and receive affection, how to set limits, how to control behaviour. Or this may go on to role playing, with the therapist perhaps playing different roles even during one session; for example, parent, teacher, friend, negotiator, demonstrator, administrator and so on. When the therapist actually takes over the role of a family member, being perhaps the child, or the father, a degree of empathy is needed, and some therapists may find this feeling difficult to achieve. However, when the real family member can accept that the therapist is really feeling himself into his situation he may then be able to try out being more positive or aggressive − or indeed the more tender and affectionate − father. These efforts will then be reinforced by the approval of the therapist (Liberman,[6] Bandura[7]).

In some families, rather than modelling for a family member the therapist may change roles with him, and invite that family member to become the therapist, even exchanging with a number of family members.

## Howells

His approach is different in that he offers a comprehensive family psychiatric service for diagnosis and treatment. Either the child is accepted as the referred patient and from the start 'the psychiatrist gives the rest of the family equal attention in his assessments and moves to treating the family as a whole (child and family psychiatry) or a family member of any age, part of the family, or the whole family is accepted for treatment (family psychiatry).'

## Child and family psychiatry (Howells[11])

In order to determine whether the 'patient' has an emotional disorder or some other clinical entity, it is usual for the psychiatrist to see both the child and the parents at the first interview, to conduct a physical and a neurological examination where necessary, and to arrange for further investigations, psychological tests and a 'play diagnosis' with the psychotherapist. These assessments are speedily carried out and the psychiatrist is able to make a formulation and a plan for treatment.

The child has individual sessions with the psychotherapist, but in most cases also takes part in family group sessions with the psychiatrist; one or other parent may also have individual sessions in addition to the group. In addition 'vector therapy' is carried out by the social worker.

## B. Variations on Family Therapy

### *Flexibility*

Family therapy can be very flexible. The setting may vary from the doctor's consulting room to family home whether it be a caravan, a council house or a mansion. The time may vary; it is usually 1½ hours, but may be as little as 1 hour or as much as 3 days; the interval between sessions may be as little as 1 week (unusual) or as much as 3 months.

### *Marathon sessions: multiple impact therapy*

In multiple impact therapy the family receives the entire attention of a team of therapists for 3 days or for a weekend. It is used particularly by Satir[5] and by the University of Texas team (McGregor *et al.*[8]). It is thought to be useful in families where the interest in and motivation for therapy is not high, for such families are more likely to attend for a 'block' session than for three weekly meetings. It is also valuable as a diagnostic and therapeutic technique with adolescent problems.

### *Multiple family therapy**

This is interesting in that it brings together two or more families who are 'strangers' to each other, and combines some of the facets of group and family therapy.

### *Co-Therapist(s)*

Advantages are that the therapy is not likely to be interfered with because of the defences of the therapists since these are likely to cancel each other out. Over-reactions and under-reactions are less likely, systems in the family which are preventing communication are more readily broken up, and 'taboo' material is more readily introduced. The two therapists talk together in the session and this clarifies confusions as they discuss what has been going on. If the two therapists are of the opposite sex this is thought to be particularly helpful.

*See Powell and Monahan,[9] and Blinder[10]

## C. Special Situations

### 'Problem families'

Having been deprived themselves, these parents are particularly liable to project conflicts onto children, spouses, in-laws and society. Skynner considers that some of these families are too primitive to benefit from family therapy, and may be more suited to multiple impact or vector therapy.

### Treatment of family where there is a brain-damaged child

Like all other children, the brain-damaged child reacts to family patterns of behaviour. In some families the brain-damaged child may be a stabilising factor in the family, draining off the family tensions. The minimally handicapped child is more liable to become disturbed, and he may find that his emotional growth and individual potential is subservient to the role of 'handicapped' or 'maladjusted' child.

### Use in early adolescence

In early adolescence where the child is acting out 'dangerously', family therapy may be useful especially where the parents are at variance, one cancelling out the strictness of the other, with the collusion of the adolescent.

One method (nearing behaviour therapy) has been called 'excommunication'. The child is presented with a united family front (parents, siblings, extended family) so that he has no room for manoeuvre (except to get out of the family and it is hoped he is too young and insecure to do this). There is no softening of any member until the adolescent shows a change of heart and behaviour. This also achieves a separation of parent and child roles, and the parents have an experience of successful working together which may spread to other situations and they may find a renewed enjoyment in their adolescent. It is necessary for the therapist to be available outside the sessions.

This is not so suitable for later adolescents, when the kind of family therapy used at the University of Texas or peer group therapy is more appropriate.

## D. Vector Therapy*

The rationale of this form of therapy is that there are forces playing on the family from within the family and without. Vector therapy aims at changing

*See Howells.[11,12]

these forces for the betterment of the family. In contrast to psychotherapy, vector therapy is less intense, more general and less concentrated, and the field of forces is outside the identified patient.

Change may be in direction, in intensity, in quality or in time. The change can offset forces outside the individual but within the family (involving one member, or more, or the whole family), or outside the family, (involving one individual, one agency, or the community as a whole). The ultimate is a change in the general culture (amelioration of poverty, housing).

It is clear when we study examples that vector therapy is often used without our knowing it, as in cases where Job spends less time with father with whom he feuds, and more with an uncle he gets on well with, or Jane spends half of the day in a nursery so that she is only exposed part-time to an irritable, depressed mother, or spends half the day with a placid neighbour and mother is enabled to work part-time. Or again, Nigel spends his evenings at a club where they build canoes and later go on the river with them, instead of roaming the streets with 'the gang'. Placement in a foster home or mal-adjusted schools or hostel are other forms of vector therapy, and Howells[12] stressed that such separations may be therapeutic and also prophylactic.

What is different is that vector therapy is being considered as a form of treatment in its own right. Vector therapy seems so easy that it may be 'done' without a plan, but one has to base the measures on a right emotional analysis of the family. This analysis must be understood by those dealing with the family (possibly family doctor, health visitor, district nurse, school welfare officer, social worker, etc. and in some cases probation officer and adult psychiatrist) so that liaison between them is kept up and planning consistent. Improvement in vector therapy lies in the building up of facilities which are not at present available to meet the emotional needs of children and families. Until the need is stated there will be no attempt to build up the facilities.

*Use of vector therapy*

The list given above of persons who may be involved with the family will suggest (and rightly) that many of the families who most benefit from vector therapy are the so-called 'problem families'. It is postulated that in these families the parents have difficulty in relating to two sets of parents, and defining family and generation boundaries. Conflicts thus tend to be spread over both the nuclear and the extended family, which results in further conflicts being stimulated since negative sentiments are readily projected on to in-laws for example. Polarisation readily takes place, and the normal supportive roles of the extended family are lost. In these families supplies of interest and affection are also limited especially where the struggle for existence (for money and food) is an everyday preoccupation.

*Crisis intervention* (Langsley,[13] Gorell-Barnes,[14]) often a form of vector therapy) and separation (not necessarily permanent) as well as more limited action bear fruit in these families, in diluting the problem and making it possible for the parents to function a little more adequately. Another aspect of crisis intervention needs to be considered, which tie in with Anthony's[15] observation that some families functioned better after illness. Both Erikson[16] and Caplan[17] have postulated that there may be increased motivation to learn new skills in a situation of high anxiety and especially where defence mechanisms fail. Although these writers were considering developmental hurdles, it may be that a similar process is initiated in some families by a situation such as illness or a family crisis, and that intervention at this time may augment the family's effort. The family may be susceptible to re-educative or therapeutic approaches at that time, perhaps offered on a whole-family basis and in the family home.

## E. Termination

The question of termination must be thought through in family therapy, although perhaps since so much was left for the family to do in the beginning much can be left to it in the ending. Some therapists, e.g. Satir, start with a time limit in view, perhaps six sessions, and Skynner does not reckon to go much beyond ten. Where the matter has been left more open, certain trends indicate that the family are reaching towards termination. They are treating one another as people rather than as persons fulfilling a role, they are enjoying one another, and enjoying persons outside the family; the family has in fact become less claustrophobic.

Termination is approaching when there is a sense that the family is moving on, having found that everything did not 'fall apart' when forbidden things were brought out into the open; when the needs of family members are being met rather than being syphoned off into socially acceptable patterns of behaviour. When the therapist realises that family 'homework' is increasing, and that stresses and feuds in the sessions are correspondingly less, he may lead the family towards termination.

In some cases the family and therapist may have to recognise that family patterns are not going to change, minor modifications may be the most that can be hoped for, but even here if the family can adjust actively to the things which cannot be changed, rather than accepting them passively, something has been gained. There is usually less resistance to termination in family therapy than in other forms of therapy. This may be because of the greater activity on the part of the therapist, but also on the part of the family, and the importance given to the family, even more so if it knows that it has been carrying on the therapy between meetings, perhaps with some family members acting as therapists.

The family may have surprised itself by what it has been able to do, and as therapy draws to a close they can know that they still have each other.

## Bibliography and Further Reading

Items marked * are particularly important sources. Unnumbered references provide alternative sources to the reference quoted immediately above.

*1. Skynner, A. C. R. (1969) A group-analytic approach to conjoint family therapy, *J. Child. Psychol. Psychiat.* **10**, 2, 81–106.

2. Skynner, A. C. R. (1967) Diagnosis, consultation and coordination of treatment, *Papers Given at the 23rd Child Guidance Inter-Clinic Conference*, National Association for Mental Health, London.

*3. Ackerman, N. (1966) *Treating the Troubled Family*, Basic Books, New York.

4. Ackerman, N. (1964) Prejudicial scapegoating and neutralising trends in the family group, in *Theory and Practice of Family Psychiatry* (ed. Howells, J. G.), Oliver & Boyd, Edinburgh and London (1968), p. 628.

*5. Satir, V. (1967) *Conjoint Family Therapy*, Science and Behaviour Books, Palo Alto.
Jackson, D. D. and Weakland, J. (1961) Conjoint family therapy, *Psychiatry*, **24**, 2, Suppl. 30–45.

6. Liberman, R. P. (1970) Behavioural approaches in family and couple therapy, *Am. J. Orthopsychiat.* **40**, 1, 106–118.

7. Bandura, A. (1969) *Principles of Behaviour Modification*, Holt, Rinehart & Winston, New York.

8. MacGregor, R. *et al.* (1964) *Multiple Impact Therapy with Families*, McGraw-Hill, London.

9. Powell, M. and Monahan, J. (1969) Reaching the rejects through multifamily group therapy, *Int. J. Grp. Psychother.* **19**, 35–43.

10. Blinder, M. G. *et al.* (1965) "M.C.F.T.": Simultaneous treatment of several families, *Am. J. Psychother.* **19**, 4, 559–569.

11. Howells, J. (1972) *Principles of Family Psychiatry*, Brunner-Mazel, New York.

12. Howells, J. (1963) Child/parent/separation as a therapeutic procedure, *Am. J. Psychiat.* **119**, 10, 922–926.

13. Langsley, D. G. *et al.* (1968) Family crisis therapy, *Family Process* **7**, 2, 145–158.

14. Gorrell-Barnes, G. (1973) Working with the family group, *Social Work Today* **4**, 3, 65–70.

15. Anthony, E. J. (1970) The mutative impact of serious mental and physical illness in a parent on family life, in *The Child in his Family*, (eds. Anthony, E. J. and Koupernik, C.), Wiley Interscience, New York.
16. Erikson, E. H. (1959) *Identity and the Life Cycle*, Psychological Issues, Monograph 1, International Universities Press, New York.
17. Caplan, G. (1964) *Principles of Preventive Psychiatry*, Tavistock Publications, London.

### PART VI

# Residential Placement

*Broadly, children are placed in residential establishments because they cannot be cared for adequately in their own homes, when there is a need to change the life base of the child. There is a lack of fit at home, when either the needs of the child are too great, their demands too exacting, or the home is in some way inadequate. Alternatively there may be some fault or lack in the provision external to the home, such as lack of day schools dealing with handicapped pupils of different kinds (including maladjusted children). Yet again, some parents elect to send their children away to schools which they consider offer more than the local provision, or simply because they seek boarding.*

---

## CHAPTER 22

## Needs and Provision

### A. Needs and Aims

What is being sought may be primarily disposal or primarily benefit. To one degree or another the residential establishment is sharing the parenting with the parents at home.

How is the placement regarded by the child and by the parents? Is he 'going away' or being 'sent away'? The latter carries a negative, defeatist and even punitive connotation, the former a positive onward-looking, even rewarding one. Yet the child of wealthy parents may be 'going' to an expensive public school because he doesn't fit in at home, because there isn't room for him in his parents' lives, or simply because they have not stopped to consider whether the placement, traditional in the family, is really suited to him. He

221

may, in fact, be as reluctant to depart as the child from a deprived home who is being 'sent away' because he has become delinquent. In families where there is no tradition of boarding there is often a feeling of failure and disgrace, and doubts and suspicions about the placement itself, and fears that the child will see it as a rejection. If the facilities can be seen to meet the needs of the child the attitude of parents and child will gradually change.

Although general provision is made, the aim must be different for each individual since for each child the kind of healthy development which can be achieved and the damage which cannot altogether be undone is different. He needs 'to be able to continue his individual development at whatever level is possible for him without such stress (or handicap) as to disable him or to overload the people with whom he lives, or to drive him into serious conflict with the community or alienation from it.' (Balbernie([1])).

Thus the residential unit has to make a reliable but constantly modifiable selection of a given range of provision for each child. The establishment needs to be able to hold the child there, but mere holding (or care) is not enough, some form of 'nurturing' is often needed, and also the maintenance and development of personality, integration and personal integrity.

It has been considered that many of the children have an 'ego handicap' and that provision has to be made for 'ego building'. Beedell([2]) thinks of residential 'treatment' as occurring within the new 'life space' provided by the establishment, and that there needs to be specialisation of task for particular residential units and careful assessment and selection. A balance has to be achieved between the insulation which is required for treatment/therapy, and rehabilitation which involves the outside, since the aim is 'after a period of time to enable children to return to their families, to other life bases or to an independent base' (Balbernie([1])). Work with parents or other persons or agencies concerned with providing a life space for the child before and after placement has to be appropriately planned and shared.

Preparation of the child for placement involves recognition of the feelings of both the child and the (failed) therapist. The decision to place away must not be seen as a reason to see the child less often, or to alter the mode of communication with the child; pre-care, care, holiday-care and after-care must be seen as continuous. The child (and also the parents) will have phantasies about the placement based on his own experience. If both parents and child can accept that he needs emotional space in which to grow, a kind of contract can be made which must be reviewed from time to time. There is a danger of home and school being split off, partly because of the 'insulation' necessary for treatment, partly because of fears (of both child and parents) of the home and school coming together, and because of ambivalence in the parents towards change in the child.


## B. Facilities

The White Paper of 1965, *The Child, the Family and the Young Offender*,[3] led the way to a new appraisal of the aims and means of placing children away from their own homes. Some but not all of its suggestions were incorporated in the Children and Young Persons Act 1969.[4] The main theme was that the decision with regard to placement should fit the needs of the child rather than his behaviour, and did away with the lumping together of all children who had committed the same 'crime' and who therefore received the same punishment; indeed it was hoped that the idea of punishment would be done away with altogether, and replaced by the idea of positive therapy. The failure or inadequacies or culpabilities of the parents were to be seen also only in relation to the needs of the child.

The hope expressed in the White Paper was that Juvenile Courts would be replaced by Family Councils whereby the parents and their child would meet together informally and in private with those persons having knowledge of their child, and with information to give, e.g. doctors, teachers, social workers and others. There would be opportunities for questions and discussion, and it was expected that the final recommendation would be seen in a positive light. This idea was not incorporated in the final form of the Act, but the way was left open for liaison between the police and those persons mentioned above in order to prevent unnecessary appearances of children at the Juvenile Courts.

One far-reaching change is that whereas previously magistrates could make 'approved school orders' indicating that in their view the young person required a particular kind of treatment, under the new act they may only make 'care orders' which leaves it up to the Director of Social Services to decide on placement, which might even be placement (under supervision) back in the child's own home, for being 'in care' does not inevitably mean 'residential' care, even where residential placement had been specifically recommended.

Although from January 1971 there is no legal distinction between the approved school system and the remainder of the child care system, and all establishments are known as 'community homes', the ex-approved schools, with their structure and expertise in dealing with children with special needs, were expected to continue to receive such children. However, whereas previously the schools were required to accept the children sent to them they are now able to pick and choose, to refuse to accept and to refuse to keep children. This has meant that they have been able to develop the sort of community they want but it has also meant that many of the most deprived, disturbed and delinquent children now find their way to the ex-children's homes, which as we shall see are poorly equipped to receive them. Prior to placement children may be sent to an assessment centre (whether they have been before the court or not) to determine the appropriate placement, which may or may not be residential. This could involve some form of intermediate treatment (with the child often residing at his own home) or placement in a community home, in-patient unit, maladjusted school or other establishment. A specific establishment is usually sought although, as we have seen, the child may appear unacceptable to the establishment approached.

It will be useful to look at the way in which approved schools, children's homes and maladjusted homes have functioned in the past and how they are functioning today.

The maladjusted schools (under education departments) were considered to have a therapeutic aim, the children's homes to provide substitute 'care' and often to 'rescue' children, while the approved schools aimed at a custodial, corrective and (hopefully) therapeutic regime. However, some maladjusted schools valued containment and structure more than some approved schools, and some 'good' children's homes or even a 'good' cottage in a not-so-good children's home were more therapeutic than either of the other two. However, some establishments did exemplify the stereotype. Some approved schools, for instance, usually of large size, perpetuated with their hierarchical structure the punitive and repressive measures, and the vicious subculture so vividly described by Wills.([5])

Allocation of children to the different establishments never really depended solely on the 'crime' (behaviour). We saw how middle-class children who stole found themselves at the clinic, while lower-class 'thieves' were more likely to land up in court. Similarly middle-class children were more likely to go to maladjusted schools, and lower-class children referred to one of the 'coercive' services, to approved schools or possibly to children's homes.

Since the 1965 White Paper very few children appear in court. By liaison via police to the agencies it is hoped to provide what is needed in the way of treatment and care, including the facilities available under 'Intermediate treatment'. Where the problem is more complex the child may be sent to an assessment centre for a period of observation and study. Families in which children are thought to be 'at risk' may be offered help by the Social Service

Department. In all these ways, with less prejudice and more fairly than in the past, an attempt is made to assess the need. Scarcity of resources and suitable placements have made implementation difficult.

## Community homes

Those which were previously children's homes seem to be in the most difficult position, whether run by local authorities or by charitable organisations. They have to cater for children who are going to spend the whole of their young lives in the home, but also for those who spend only a short time, or who are 'in and out'. They have to care for individual children, or for a whole family of children, for children whose parents are completely out of the picture and for others where the parents visit regularly or spasmodically.

They have constant staff shortages, both in quantity and quality. Some staff members are drawn to the work because they were themselves brought up in a children's home, others because of problems of their own. They seek satisfaction for themselves in their work; some by identifying with the children succeed quite well since by caring for the children they are caring for themselves, but others feel in a situation of sibling rivalry with their charges and cannot be objective or allow the children's needs. Many feel readily rejected by the child, who may be in his turn projecting the feelings he has for his parents onto the houseparents, and they feel resentful towards the real parents who 'let the child down' by not writing, not visiting or by breaking promises, but are still wanted by the child. Among the staff may be older unmarried women (it has been remarked that spinsters are among the more stable members of staff) with unlimited time and devotion to give, couples who may have families of their own, and others will be young men or women hardly more than children themselves emotionally. It is essential that these people learn to get on together, for it is fatal if staff dissension or jealousies present the child with a picture which is already too familiar to him (Burmeister[6]).

Dedication and a common purpose may achieve the harmony needed, but understanding and training are also essential. Claire Winnicott[7] has written 'The care of these children does require a teamwork approach so that the stress is shared between a group of people who know what they are about and who consciously seek to provide together the human reliability and human care that is needed.' This cannot be replaced by subjectivity and dedication, which tend to lead to an attitude where staff feel that they should be able to manage all children and all situations and feel they have failed if they cannot. One of the nation-wide charitable organisations set up a unit to which branches could refer problem children for advice or for treatment. Referrals were so few that 90 percent of the children in the unit were referred by local authorities, yet all the branches had disturbed children. Similar denial results when a suggestion is made to transfer a child from one family cottage to another. This does not allow for variation in the capabilities of the house-parents, some of whom may cope well with small children but have problems with adolescents or vice versa. So long as one house is not made a ragbag for the misfits from all the other houses, it seems practical to make the best use of people's talents and feelings of jealousy or failure are inappropriate. So flexibility, selection and specialisation are required.

Now that the 'stigma' of the approved school is removed and all Homes are Community Homes, establishments functioning as children's homes, especially those with a reputation for handling difficult children and accepting challenges, have been flooded with deprived, immature, disturbed and delinquent children, who have been sent to them from assessment centres. Since the homes do not have the requisite increase in number and quality of staff, some of these children have to be moved on resulting in further damage to them.

### Approved schools (Community homes, social service department)

Some of the children who would have been placed in approved schools are now 'tried out' in maladjusted schools or children's homes, but there remains a need for establishments to cater for certain kinds of disturbed and delinquent children and adolescents. As we saw in regard to delinquency a variety of regimes are required and the hope is that these will gradually be provided and the methods and the results scientifically studied.

At present at many of the 'homes' the large size without subdivision except possibly into (still large) 'houses' and the low staff/pupil ratio with retention of the hierarchical structure slow down progress. A few 'homes' have set up true therapeutic communities with favourable staff/pupil ratios, with adequate facilities and with psychiatric help, but these can cater for only a few.

### Schools for the maladjusted (Education department)

Local Education Authorities set up their own maladjusted schools providing 'treatment in an educational setting', and hostels (education at local schools, though many have a hostel class also). They also sponsor children at independent maladjusted schools, and also to a lesser degree at schools not specifically catering for the maladjusted but which take a proportion of disturbed children, though in these there is often a higher proportion of these children than the numbers sponsored by Local Education Authorities would suggest. In addition some authorities have boarding places attached to day schools (these have usually been grammar schools, but this is changing) and where such places are not available may send a child to a hostel for maladjusted children from which the child attends a local school.

These sorts of provision usually meet a social need for children who are not seriously maladjusted. 'Good' education authorities are generous both in their own provision and in using other facilities. This introduces the whole spectrum of boarding schools, for those supposedly catering for 'normal' children from 'normal' homes find themselves (and not only the 'progressive' ones) catering for numbers of children who are disturbed. Many children are sent to these schools because of family tradition or social aspirations, but without regard to the suitability for the particular child. Some go off (to preparatory schools) at a young age and a number of these become disturbed. Others go because they are already showing maladjustment or because the home is breaking up, or parents going abroad; some of the latter become maladjusted. Schools with a reputation for being good at dealing with 'problems' may become overloaded with such children.

## C. An Overview of Boarding

S. Millham([8],[9]) has looked at all types of residential schools (including approved schools old and new, but not children's homes) and criticises them broadly as being irrelevant to living in the community outside.

He considers them to be too total, claustrophobic and narrow. The schools and the children are isolated from the outside because of custodial or protective needs, the outside doesn't come inside, and the inside doesn't go outside. Within the school a little world is set up, and both staff and children feel 'we have everything here'. Many children become 'indoctrinated' and bear the 'stamp' of the school, and the school may bear the 'stamp' of the 'head'. There is too much public and too little private living, and a denial of rich emotional life for the pupils while the school pays lip service to the needs of the growing child. In many schools staff problems and organisation become fossilised, with increasing power of certain masters, and the children react by identity and conformity, or by withdrawal and more rarely rebellion (these usually leave). In this situation scapegoating by the peer group is easily developed and hidden. Millham considers that many of the school heads are arrogant, often with an evangelical mission or with a romantic idea of the role of the school itself.

A corollary of all this is that as the inside (school) becomes more important, the outside (the family) become less important. Parents are often shuffled aside, particularly those who have already been defined as inadequate, and the ideals of the school are often very different from parental values. The schools may disregard the hopes and expectations of the parents, who tend to be blamed (by their children too) for not 'seeing the point'.

Clearly all this is less likely to happen when the parents are paying the fees, since to some extent they can 'call the tune', but they may also be or may become identified with the school culture or, if not, may be unable to break through the web of power tradition. The parents, like the children, have to follow the school rules and regulations about all sorts of minor details, are made to feel a nuisance if they ask for 'special arrangements', and 'interfering' if they express worries about their child. If they persist it becomes clear that they are 'not wanted' by the school. For them, as for the children, it is much simpler to conform.

Millham recognises that boarding schools do have a role to play, especially in emerging adolescents who are having difficulties. The schools can recognise the adolescent role (with eventual improvement in the behaviour of the pupil); they can reduce pressure, they can share the child's problems by discussion singly or in groups, they can remotivate the child. (Some adolescent boys as a result become closer to their fathers, but tend to become alienated from their mothers.) Many of these adolescents develop a high level of commitment to the schools and find it hard to leave, returning often. This is seen by the schools as evidence of their success.

## D. Rejects of the Residential System

Residential placement often denotes or is felt to denote a failure in some other provision, e.g. child guidance treatment. Yet there are children who fail in or who are rejected by one residential establishment after another. These have been called the 'residual/residual' population. What is the appropriate placement for them, something quite different from what is already provided, or can it be provided within existing establishments using new concepts or methods of approach?

Many of this residual/residual group are older adolescents, usually male, who have shown particularly difficult and disturbed behaviour in approved schools (now community homes) or in-patient units (they have often had to be transferred to adult wards). The Home Office in conjunction with the Department of Health has set up one unit in which psychiatric treatment is available both for 'patients' and for counselling staff.

## E. In-Patient Units

Many of these are attached to psychiatric hospitals, although the buildings stand apart, and often some distance from the main hospital. A few are purpose-built and some of these are independent of a psychiatric hospital. They may be staffed wholly or partly from the parent hospital; a few are staffed separately. There is usually a favourable patient/staff ratio, and the staff will include some specialist workers according to the orientation of the child psychiatrist. Units may be for pre-adolescents, young adolescents, or older adolescents; they may be one-sex or mixed.

Units vary according to the kind of problem they take and most have their own special flavour or atmosphere. Those catering for younger children may develop an interest in autism or children with organic factors or developmental disorders. Some units taking older children prefer anxious, neurotic patients, or children with psychosomatic disorders, and find the aggressive or 'acting out' children difficult to handle in the units they have set up. Those taking the more extroverted children often lean heavily on the parent hospital, as do those which include severely disturbed adolescents, perhaps early schizophrenics. Most of these units regard themselves as geared to investigations, assessment and short-term treatment, and also research. They are therefore of limited use for children who require long-term placement.

The need for places in hospital units is not met by the supply, neither in number nor in kind of provision. The needs of the most difficult and disturbed children are not any more adequately met in the hospital units than in the maladjusted schools, and Warren considers that the needs of these children have 'scarcely been considered'.

Most units cater for children under the age of 12, and there are few units for older adolescents. In total there were eighteen units for adolescents in 1969. Most older seriously disturbed adolescents were still being admitted to adult psychiatric wards. The need is for different kinds of units for adolescents of different ages, level of sophistication and problems.

Bibliography and Further Reading

Items marked * are particularly important sources. Unnumbered references provide alternative sources to the references quoted immediately above.

*1.  Balbernie, R. (1966) *Residential Work with Children*, Pergamon Press, Oxford.
*2.  Beedell, C. (1970) *Residential Life with Children*, Routledge & Kegan Paul, London.
  3.  *The Child, The Family and the Young Offender* (1965) H.M.S.O., London.
  4.  The Childrens and Young Persons Act 1969. H.M.S.O., London.
  5.  Wills, W. D. (1971) *Spare the Child*, Penguin Educational Special, Penguin Books, Harmondsworth.
  6.  Burmeister, E. (1960) *The Professional Houseparent*, Columbia University Press, New York.
  7.  Winnicott, C. (1963) Face to face with children, in *New Thinking for Changing Needs*, Association of Social Workers, Dennison House, London.
      Morrison, R. L. (1967) The idea of therapeutic communities, in *New Thinking about Institutional Care*, Association of Social Workers, Dennison House, London.
  *   Dockar-Drysdale, B. (1968) *Therapy in Child Care*, Longmans, London.
      Winnicott, D. W. (1965) *The Maturational Processes and the Facilitating Environment*, Hogarth Press, London.
  8.  Millham, S., Lambert, R. and Bullock, R. (1974) *A Chance of a Lifetime – an Overview of Boarding Schools (Boys and Coeducational)* Weidenfeld & Nicoloson (in press).
  9.  Millham, S., Bullock, R. and Cherrett, P. (1974) *After Grace – Teeth – Approved Schools*, Chaucer Press, London.
  *   Stroud, J. (ed.) (1973) *Services for Children and their Families*, Pergamon Press, Oxford.

## CHAPTER 23

# Treatment, the Role of the Child Psychiatrist

Two aspects of treatment in residential establishments concern us, the effect of the total environment on the disturbed child, and the specific therapies, individual or group, which may be carried out by the child psychiatrist or by members of the staff.

In my view the role of the child psychiatrist who visits a maladjusted school should be different from his role as consultant to a community home. In the school most of the children will be suffering from neurotic-type disorders, and individual or group psychotherapy along the lines already described is indicated. The school will be run to a greater or less degree as a therapeutic community, and the staff, often with a background in teaching, usually have a special interest, (and often special training) in the disturbed child. They need some help to deepen their understanding of particular problems (but not necessarily over particular children). Certain schools cater for a particular type of child, for example the affectionless child, or children who have organically-determined problems, but in these cases the school is set up in a special way, and the staff have a particular orientation and training.

In regard to community homes Millham([1]) found in the ex-approved school a highly disturbed component, to the degree of 1:4, and many of these have a fair proportion of mature and trained staff, and provide a structured environment. Some have branched away, for example, the Cotswold Community and Peper Harow, and have special community and therapeutic regimes. Classification and assessment centres allocate children to particular community homes, and in time the difference between individual community homes will depend less on previous function than on the internal planning and allocation of children to it.

## Community Homes

The following remarks apply particularly to ex-children's homes now functioning in their new role and taking in increased numbers of difficult and disturbed children, but with poor staffing ratios.

*Helping the staff to meet the needs of the child*

The role of the child psychiatrist is often viewed as being directed solely towards the individual child, who is too difficult, disturbed or handicapped for the staff to handle alone. As the head of one approved school for girls put it, 'We can't get through to this disruptive rebellious child, some sessions with you may help her to unwind.'

The idea is to hand over the child, who now becomes a patient, to the child psychiatrist, so that he may be changed and rendered more acceptable, or so that the staff be advised how to handle him. Failing this they hope an alternative placement may be suggested. Meanwhile the institution can carry on just as before.

We have noted that children appear differently to different people, yet in the community home the person who comes each week to the psychiatrist to report progress (or more often regress) of the child is the very person who has found him too difficult to handle. Other people who come into contact with him during the whole day may have quite a different picture of him. The idea of a 'context profile', as outlined by B. Dockar-Drysdale,([2]) is that all persons dealing with a particular child during the 24 hours, pool not so much their observations but their experiences of that child in order to learn about him and perhaps see him with new eyes. Or the different 'times' in the day can be pooled to form a composite picture; getting up, going to bed, mealtimes, playtimes, in between times, special times. Going to sleep when the child has to surrender himself to unconsciousness, to the unknown; and waking, and getting up when he has to face the reality of another day are the hardest times for a disturbed child, and mealtimes are said to be a mirror of family life. The context profile is most suited to a total set up with home and school on the same premises, but a variant may be mounted in a home where children go out to school. All the adults who have had dealings with the child during a 24-hour period meet together for 1½ hours. For a child of secondary school age this may involve several teachers, dinner ladies, sports coach and others from school, all the people who have been involved with him in the home and during recreation or in between times. As they describe and discuss, relate and interpret, each adult gains an overall picture of the child much freer than usual of bias, prejudice and false impressions. The participating and listening adults learn something about themselves as well as about the child, and often about the total situation in class, school or home. However reluctant or critical initially, the participants end by agreeing unanimously that the meeting has been fruitful, and beyond its usefulness for that particular child.

This kind of meeting often leads to the staff of the home wanting to know more about the needs of the children, and how they have come to be as they are. In-service training, even if they have received it, often does not prepare them for the severe problems they meet. Nearly all the children have known some deprivation and many traumatic experiences. They arrive at the home with a basic distrust of human relationships, have great difficulty in making them, are culturally deprived and have problems in communication especially on the verbal side. Some children will have lacked 'primary experience', others will have been partially deprived. They can only be helped by provision in the present of what they have lacked in the past, and when this has been achieved by gradual correction of their distrust of human relationships. They need stable supplies from one or more members of staff, who may themselves need considerable support from the psychiatrist while giving this; and this is a more worthwhile job for him than seeing children who are often too frozen, suspicious or frightened to respond to him, except on a very long-term basis, for the psychiatrist may be seen as yet another threatening person who has power over the child's life (Winnicott,[3,4] Klein and Riviere[5]).

The most deprived require an opportunity to retrace their steps by regression before they can progress. This can perhaps be done by making one person available to the child at a particular time each day in a place where he can be as babyish as he pleases. Difficulties may be put in the way of doing something like this, partly because a distinction has not been made between 'function' and 'role'. Workers in a community home have functions such as 'housemother', 'cook' and 'handyman', to which they must adhere to give security and structure, but within these functions there is room for them to play different roles to different children at different times. The time spent does not have to be long; 10 minutes each night or an hour a week may be sufficient, nor does a complicated plan have to be made. One housemother spent just 10 minutes each evening with one deprived boy, while they sat together in a special low chair in an alcove off a corridor and looked at a picture book together. In some cases it may be necessary for someone else to take over the 'function' temporarily, such as relieving the cook for half an hour while she gives a teenage boy his 'ration' of love.

An alternative is setting up a cottage, or part of a house or building where a group of children (some of whom may be adolescents of 14 or 15) live with two or more adults. While 'at home' nutritive supplies and comforts of all kinds are available. A flexible school regime combines with this best, though some children are able to take a full day's school after a time, living as it were two lives. 'Weaning' from this home has to be gradual. The slightly better integrated children may have started off with adequate experiences, but since have been exposed to frightening and disturbing experiences, buffeted from pillar to post, and some find that the strain of adjusting to a new school as well as to a new home drains away their slender resources. They may run away or become delinquent, and because of their behaviour they are in danger of being rejected yet again and moved on. Yet their great need is for a permanent home. It is necessary to look beneath the outward behaviour to the fear, distrust and despair.

It is instructive to study a particular aspect of behaviour of children in community homes, particularly one which causes concern, such as destructive behaviour. Soon after arrival disturbed children will do damage to home property, to themselves and to their clothes. It has been suggested that if opportunities are taken from them to do this (such as the home being too grand, or the punishments too severe) the child is not able to work through this phase and reach a point of wishing to make restitution. Mrs Drysdale found that boys break more, but girls tear up more; but both sexes make restitution by doing jobs, decorating, growing vegetables, or making presents, sometimes for the person they have damaged, sometimes for the community.

Both the unintegrated children who have begun to respond and the slightly more integrated children need opportunities for ego-strengthening experiences and for forming and testing relationships. 'Function' and 'role' are important here too and attention to bedtimes and getting up times.

Children who have been repeatedly let down by their parents and others are wary and suspicious of new overtures, and it is most important that staff realise the importance of being behind the child, and not letting him down, which is not the same thing as failing him unavoidably by being ill, going on holiday, or having a day off. Not letting down means doing things that all good enough parents do, such as seeing that the child has the right clothing and equipment, baking a cake for the school 'bring and buy', going to 'open days', giving support, showing interest and responding to the child's cues. One headmaster commented that only the children from the 'home' were unable to buy the photographs taken of each child at school. When he mentioned it to the superintendent, the reply was 'It isn't worth it'.

Trust can only develop gradually; in the meantime these children can be helped by play opportunities, made freely available to them without direction from an adult who is present merely to facilitate; painting materials, clay, puppets, dolls, dressing up things, masks, simple building kits, cars, balsa blocks are all suitable.

*Helping the staff with their own roles**

Immature staff who have been deprived themselves may need to grow and mature as the children do. In addition problems arise because of the dual role which the residential worker has to fulfil. She (or he) is expected to keep a clean and tidy house, yet a homely one, to observe overall standards and discipline imposed from above (which may be contrary to her own ideas), yet be a parent to the children, to preserve the 'image' of the home to the outside world and yet allow the children to 'have fun' when they go out. The worker is rarely told about things which parents would normally know about, she is rarely consulted about plans or decisions. She has to share the child with the natural parents, with people higher in the home hierarchy, with the school and probably with the field worker.

It was a move in the right direction when one large voluntary organisation decided to do away with the position of 'nurse' in their large branches. Her work, of treating minor ailments, taking children to hospital, is now taken care of by the house 'parent'. This raises the question of whether some home visiting should be done by the residential worker rather than the field worker. Shortage of staff would probably preclude this in most establishments, and would probably also be resisted by the field worker who regards the child as her 'client' rather than seeing her role as supporting and helping the family while the child is away.

Finally the residential worker may feel discouraged, for while she sees herself having to cope with more disturbed and deprived children than ever before, she is aware that 'quality' staff are attracted to work in smaller 'therapeutic' units, maladjusted schools or in-patient units. She may envy the field worker who has the positive aim of keeping children in their own homes or in foster homes.

The field worker however has problems of her own (Winnicott([7])). It is usually she who brings the child to the home in the first place, and she may feel a sense of failure in so doing as this step was to be avoided except as a last resort. This may lead her to make promises (like the 'guilty' parents) about visiting which it is impossible for her to keep, and when she does visit

*See Burmeister. ([6])

she may feel a coldness from some of the staff so that working together is not always achieved. Both child and staff may blame her for parental visits or promises about home leave which have not been kept, and the child may turn from her and lean towards the residential worker, or he may cling to her since she represents his family and the 'outside' but make demands which she cannot meet. When she attends case conferences at the Home, and is unable to make on-the-spot decisions without consulting her superiors she may be blamed and thought of as 'useless'. She may indeed feel this as she may not be readily available to the child and the home in times of crisis. It may be that the role of the field worker in relation to community homes should be re-examined.

The child psychiatrist may find it hard to escape the role of the 'expert' who 'treats' the child (Lavery and Stone[8]). He may feel frustrated when his advice, for example that a child is not yet ready to face a full day at school, is not taken, or he is not consulted about moving a disturbed child from one house to another, to give two examples from my own experience. Other suggestions about possible changes or innovations fall on deaf ears, and suggestions about group discussions with staff may be ignored. Even treatment of the 'patient', if not along the lines envisaged by the head, may be sabotaged. In the approved school for girls already mentioned I had a regular weekly therapy group with some of the girls. One week the secretary was instructed to telephone me to announce, 'We shall not be having the therapy *class* this week as the girls are going to the cinema'.

It seems that the staff do not feel safe unless the psychiatrist keeps to his prescribed role, and it behoves him to hurry slowly and to show his realisation of the very real difficulties under which the staff do a tremendously good job, and to recognise the fear behind the resistance that psychiatric 'gimmicks' might unleash dangerous forces and worsen the situation.

### Bibliography and Further Reading

Items marked * are particularly important sources. Unnumbered references provide alternative sources to the references quoted immediately above.

\*      Bowlby, J. (1970) *Child Care and the Growth of Love,* Penguin Books, Harmondsworth.

1.     Millham, S., Bullock, R. and Cherrett, P. (1974) *After Grace – Teeth – Approved Schoools,* Chaucer Press, London.

2. Dockar-Drysdale, B. (1968) *Therapy in Child Care*, Longmans, London.
3. Winnicott, D. W. (1952) Psychoses and child care, in *Collected Papers* (1958), Tavistock Publications, London.
4. Winnicott, D. W. (1960) Ego distortion in terms of true and false self, in *Therapeutic Consultations in Child Psychiatry* (1971), Hogarth Press and the Institute of Psychoanalysis, London.
5. Klein, M. and Riviere, J. (1938) *Love, Hate and Reparation*, Hogarth Press, London.
6. Burmeister, E. (1960) *The Professional Houseparent*, Columbia University Press, New York.
7. Winnicott, C. (1964) Casework and agency function, in *Child Care and Social Works*, Codicote Press, London.
8. Lavery, L., and Stone, F. H. (1965) Psychotherapy of a deprived child, *J. Child. Psychol. Psychiat.* **6**, 2, 115–124.

### PART VII

# Winds of Change

---

## CHAPTER 24

## The Future of Child Psychiatry

Although it is not yet clear what the future holds for child psychiatry it appears that the final proposals of the Secretary of State will retain it as a specialist service with a consultant child psychiatrist as director of a multi-disciplinary team. Yet although the more flexible working arrangements suggested in the DES/DHSS([1]) draft circulars match the trend shown already in clinics, where not every member of the team is involved with every case, it is hoped that the 'network of services' envisaged will not disrupt the working clinical teams. It is to be deplored if the stress laid on hospital-based clinics and units means that child guidance clinics based on the community are to be regarded as an inferior service. Both hospital-based and community-based clinics are dealing with similar child psychiatric problems, and they should be regarded as complementary parts of a unified service.

The name child guidance does perhaps carry a somewhat old-fashioned, though respectable, image, and it may be that a move to call both types of clinics by the same name is overdue. Possible titles would be Child Psychiatric, or Child and Family Psychiatric Clinic.

Other likely changes follow trends which are already clear, such as a move towards a child psychiatry which has closer links with medical centres and with the community. There may be more hospital-based clinics, and more clinics attached to health centres, with relatively few in the kind of buildings which house them at present. Child psychiatrists will increase the time spent in paediatric departments, but also in assessment centres (mainly under social services) and community homes. The child psychiatrist, if working in a 'teaching area', will be employed by the area health authority, but if working in other hospitals or clinics, by the regional health authority.

The employment arrangements for psychologists (educational and clinical) are not likely to change. They will continue to be seconded to child guidance clinics by their education department, but their consultative role, already developing, is likely to be extended. It will still be based on collaboration and consultation with the other members of the 'team' but will have more autonomy.

Two factors leave the position of the social worker in some doubt. Previously seconded full-time to child guidance by the health (or in some cases by the education) department of the local authority, he will in future come under the large umbrella of the social service department (or possibly education department if at present he is so employed). Moreover, following recommendations of the *Committee on Local Authority and Allied Personal Social Services* of 1968 (Seebohm),([2]) social workers are to receive a 'generic' training, which will prepare them for a wide variety of social work in the community. The aim is that one worker will be responsible for all aspects of the health of a family, rather than there being a division among a number of social workers.

It is in connection with the social worker as a member of the clinic team that the greatest changes are likely to occur, and the uncertain effect of this on child guidance (and child psychiatric) clinics and on the social work profession itself has given cause for concern and raises a number of questions.*

Will the social worker be seconded full-time and permanently to child guidance or will 'nominal sessions' in the social service department form the thin end of a very large wedge, so that he finds himself with increasing duties in that department, as part of the area team and with perhaps a personal case-load? Will there continue to be a 'psychiatric' social worker with the sort of training and skills outlined on page 144.

It appears that some university departments at least will continue to offer specialist training, and part of the training will be field work in clinics where presumably psychiatric social workers will still be available as supervisors. To

---

*The definitive circular 3/74([3]) (Department of Education and Science, Department of Health and Social Security and Welsh Office([4])) comes down firmly on a medical model for child guidance with child psychiatrists working both in hospitals and the community in a flexible way with colleagues of different disciplines. The 'network of services' is again stressed along with pooling of resources, the team approach is seen as useful in carrying out the combined approach required by families.

change this would be likely to lower the status and working of the social work profession as a whole, and of child psychiatry in particular.

It is unlikely that the social worker could continue to provide the long-term skilled 'casework' so essential in work in the clinic if competing demands from other parts of the service become too great. It is not important what the social worker is called, whether 'generic', 'psychiatric' or 'medical' but the kind of training he experiences and the kind of work he does and is allowed to do is paramount.

It is expected that non-medical psychotherapists and behaviour therapists will have a greater part to play in clinic teams in the future.

## Bibliography and Further Reading

1.   Department of Education and Science Draft Circular, 1973, London.
2.   *Report of the Committee on Local Authority and Allied Personal Social Services* 1968, (The Seebohm Report), H.M.S.O., London.
3.   Department of Education and Science Circular 3/74, London.
4.   Department of Health and Social Security, Welsh Office, Cardiff.

## CHAPTER 25

# The Child Psychiatrist Present and Future

## New Roles for the Child Psychiatrist

### 1. In children's wards, with paediatrician and nursing staff

In the paediatric ward, as in the children's home, the role of the child psychiatrist was seen to be limited to examining individual children who were thought to have some 'psychiatric overlay' (whatever that may mean) or to collaborate with the management of a psychosomatic condition, or perhaps more recently to advise on a suspected case of 'battering'.

Paediatricians vary in their willingness to accept a child psychiatrist as a colleague. Some, who may be thought of as 'psychiatric paediatricians', may welcome the opportunity for the discussion of common interests, but may also resent the psychiatrist, unconsciously wishing themselves in his shoes. Others, neuro-paediatricians or paediatric physicians, may resist the psychiatric approach, especially the psycho-dynamic approach. The child psychiatrist must accept both attitudes. Although initially the first may seem easier to work with, hidden snags may appear, and in fact, if the psychiatrist is able to show himself to be flexible and useful on the children's ward, or in the out-patient department, he may be able to work out a very fruitful collaboration with paediatricians of the second type.

Nurses also follow the two main categories: those who embrace the purely physical standpoint, and those who are 'interested' in the psychological approach. Their training and assignment to a particular consultant also affects their orientation. It is easy to see why nurses may feel safer with the more measurable and understandable physical methods of treatment. Nevertheless the sphere in which the child psychiatrist can be most useful is working with the nursing staff. Examples might be collaborating with them over cases of encopresis, anorexia nervosa or obesity. A number of different techniques, such as role playing, behaviour modification, nurturing therapy, or offering

242

opportunities for regression may be utilised by nurses, and indeed are often used without awareness of what is being done. This unawareness may lead to arbitrary changes or withdrawal of the therapy, or perhaps the institution of a regime in hospital which is not paralleled by home treatment.

The child psychiatrist may also help with day to day problems with the children on the ward, with the parents who visit, and with the children who have no parents visiting them — who may be in a worse position than they would have been in the days before free visiting on the children's wards. Since these 'deprived' children do not complain, their need is not always seen. At a study day involving paediatricians, child psychiatrists and nursing staff, discussion arose about the suggestion that a particular nurse should be attached to such a child. Several staff members were strongly against this, feeling that the child would become too demanding, too dependent and would show too much feeling.

The question of feeling arises particularly in incurable illness or imminent death, with a taboo on talking about the true situation to the child or to the relatives. Yet children who are deteriorating often do realise what is happening to them, and it often helps them and their families if things are brought out into the open (Anthony,[1] Woodward[2]). When this is done, some families may decide to take their child home to die, and even if they do not, each day which the family has together can be enjoyed and remembered, instead of the artificial meetings which are 'gone through' when a pretence of normality is being kept up. When the child dies, the family may proceed naturally to a joint and shared mourning which minimises the risks of the lingering problems which we saw in the case of Glen (p. 79).

When the child psychiatrist can become a well-known figure on the children's ward, part of the 'team', easy contacts may develop with other visiting specialists, and useful discussions may develop with them, either informally or at small staff gatherings, for example with surgeons, about the inadvisability of doing cold surgery on children between the ages of 3 and 5, especially where the body orifices are concerned (see Caplan,[3] Irvine[4]).

He may also work with the medical social worker, and also with the health visitor in the field with families where a child has a psychosomatic problem, or where a child shows a deprivation syndrome or suffers multiple 'accidents'.

## 2. With family doctor and health visitor

Many family doctors are alert to the needs mentioned above, for example the avoidance of non-urgent surgery in young children and other danger times for operations and separations, and the importance of helping a family who have a damaged or dying child. They may be able to assist in the support of certain inadequate families rather than advocating the removal of the children for hospitalisation or convalescence on the least provocation. It is important, however, for the child psychiatrist to keep these topics to the fore, and occasional case conferences held at the doctor's surgery or at the child guidance clinic may be most fruitful as an exercise in collaboration, and may also help each to understand better the work which the other does. Such conferences have been held recently on a case of precocious puberty in a girl aged 7, a girl of 14 with Turner's syndrome, (see p. 198) and the case of a severely phobic boy, symbiotically tied to his mother (Balint([5])).

The role of the health visitor has changed and enlarged greatly, and these workers often have the closest knowledge and contact with families. Their influence can be tremendously valuable, in an educative, counselling or modelling role. Close liaison and working together between the health visitor and the child psychiatrist may be the method of choice in some problem families, parents who cannot keep a safe home, etc; since she is often better accepted by the family through long familiarity than the social worker from the clinic or social services.

## 3. Work with teachers and in schools

In some cases it is appropriate for the child psychiatrist, perhaps in collaboration with the educational psychologist, to work directly with the school over particular problems rather than merely to see the child and family in the clinic. This could be useful in the case of children who are refusing school, or children who are about to be excluded from school, both situations which concern teachers greatly. Individual conferences of one team member (usually the psychologist) and one teacher may be less fruitful than broader meetings. The fact that the psychologist is part of the clinic team is a tremendous advantage to the team though it may cause problems for the psychologist with 'a foot in both camps'. There should not, of course, be two camps and it is up to the child psychiatrist to do everything he can to bring the parties together in a meaningful way.

The child psychiatrist may be able to help teachers towards a change in viewpoint from superficial (behaviour) orientation to dynamic (causal) orientation (Levitt,[6] Isaac,[7] Smith,[8] Irvine[4]). This does not entail passing on a ready-made interpretation from the clinic, but getting the teachers to look behind the behaviour, and to talk about it together to discover the meaning (as was done in the 'context' meeting p. 232), not to reinforce the negative view of the difficult behaviour by constant reiteration of examples, but to look for other aspects of behaviour which a child may show to certain persons or in certain situations.

As well as helping with a kind of deconditioning technique in school phobic children, the opposite technique may sometimes be used for children showing unacceptable behaviour, which may be reinforced by the attention and even the punishment given. As far as possible, this kind of behaviour should be ignored by all concerned with the child in school, but all positive effort or behaviour is praised; this may enable the child to adopt a new role among his peers as well as with his teachers. It is important to alert the home to what is being done so that they may follow a similar procedure (Meyer and Chesser[9]).

Child psychiatrists need to be aware of the phantasies which teachers may have about the clinic team and the psychologist and psychiatrist in particular (Moore [10]). When the psychologist only visits the school as part of his role as a member of the clinic team (as ambassador or liaison officer) he (or she) is most likely to arouse phantasies in teachers, but even if she goes only to carry out tests, uneasy feelings may be provoked, and defences mobilised. If the psychologist has previously been a teacher, the teachers may fear that he will compare their work with an ideal standard, or with other schools he may visit; he in his turn may envy the teachers their nutritive role as teachers, or feel guilt about having deserted this field.

Resistance may be shown by the headteacher (and others) in a number of ways, the most common of which is by assuming a dependent relationship and forcing the psychologist into an omnipotent role, which, if he accedes, colludes with the teacher's unconscious wish for dependency, but also places him in a vulnerable position since the hostility which is also present may mean that he is set insoluble problems or that the suggestions he offers are sabotaged. It is therefore important that discussions between the psychologist and the teachers are a genuine exchange with both sides contributing honestly.

The second method of resistance is by control of the psychologist's activities; he may be diverted from the aim of his visit which was perhaps to interview a class teacher or to test a child, and instead he may find himself closeted with the headteacher or testing a child in a noisy corridor. These ruses may arise if the headteacher is unsure of his position, especially with his own staff, as he may find it too threatening to allow the psychologist to discuss children with his assistants, but in most cases the teacher feels a sense of failure when he has to ask for help from the psychologist or from the clinic, unless the psychologist can be seen as a helpful colleague.

The class teacher may also become anxious, first by the referral of a child from his class, then by the removal of that child from his class for testing, and later, even more, by the regular absences of the child for treatment. He may envy the psychologist the time he is able to spend alone with the child, and even more the psychiatrist for the therapeutic relationship which develops. This may explain some of the remarks made to the professional worker or to the child or the parents.

Many of these reactions and defences effect the situation when the child psychiatrist is directly involved, whether by the teacher visiting the clinic or the psychiatrist visiting the school. Both reactions may appear: the casting of the psychiatrist in the omnipotent role (and asking him for solutions he is unable to give) and the teacher insisting on his right as head to control the situation at school. Even where explanations have been given and discussions allowed, ending with the evolution of an apparently acceptable plan, this may be forgotten or thrown overboard at a later stage, especially if the 'hot line' with the clinic is loosened as things seem to be going well. An example is a case of school refusal, where the plan is gradual introduction to school and a bolt-hole for the child within the school should he become excessively anxious. After a time the headteacher may throw aside the agreed plan, and insist on 'attendance all day, every day, at all classes or else'. This may be because of slow progress, 'snide' remarks from some members of his staff, and his own uncertainties about his omnipotent role as head of the school in respect of a child who seems to be 'getting away with it', and who may, moreover, reject his overtures and run to the arranged bolt hole.

As psychiatrists have not been accustomed to visit schools the headteacher may feel flattered, but also threatened and worried about relating to this somewhat magic figure.

If the social worker visits the school, this usually brings in the family aspect; and teachers may have to alter their child-orientated approach and look at the problems which the parents have. They are often better able to do this when there are emotional problems in the family than where the 'problem' is simply a cultural one, for example a delinquent sub-culture or an immigrant family who do not see the good of what the school is trying to do, but look only up a narrow academic alley. The social worker has often a good chance however of forming a new and more understanding link between home and school.

Probably the most fruitful way is for the whole clinic team to visit the school, rather than for the school to visit the whole team (in the clinic). The team may go about a particular child, and if this be a child who is disruptive and a severe behaviour problem of which the school wants to be rid (if not of the problem then the child) it is important that what Skynner[11] has called 'the minimum sufficient network' of persons be assembled, so that no-one can say later that he was not involved. In some cases the parents may also be invited, perhaps to a rather smaller gathering.

In other instances the discussion of a child by the whole team gives the school a much better idea of what the clinic is able to do and, even more important, what it cannot do. Or a series of more general meetings may be held, perhaps in a neutral room such as the library and at a time such as 4.30 p.m. when teachers who are interested will be able to attend. An open discussion method may be used, and although the teachers may find this threatening at first, the flexibility may enable them later to participate in a more spontaneous way than would happen in a more teaching-type setting. Or the team (or one member) may work with small teaching groups (Smith,[8] Isaac[7]).

Ancillary members of staff must not be forgotten, and those carrying out supervision during out-of-classroom periods, especially dinner breaks, would particularly benefit from some understanding in handling difficult children by methods which neither allow the sort of release which some disturbed children are unable to control, nor a rigid control which suppresses and dams up feeling.

Needless to say the co-operation of the headteacher is essential.

### 4. Limitations of out-patient therapy

A realistic appraisal has to be made of the usefulness of out-patient treatment in dealing with very disturbed and often antisocial children. Not unnaturally the more disturbed (socially deviant) a child is, the more urgently is treatment sought by those dealing with the child, teacher, parent or probation officer.

Scott states 'the indiscriminate taking on for treatment of these children in out-patient departments produces appallingly poor results' and adds that 'the supportive relationship and the interruption of a vicious circle of family tensions could equally well have been accomplished by a skilful probation officer.' He considers that the psychiatrist's role is important in diagnosis, which includes contact in order to observe response to suggested measures, and to give guidance and support to social worker or probation officer involved. He adds that in the early stages (even pre-school) he can be much more effective. In other cases psychiatric treatment is likely to have some success with individuals who have reached a certain level of personality integration. This aspect has been dealt with in the section on delinquency.

It seems important for the psychiatrist working in a clinic to face up clearly to the limitations of his role in treating those children which referring agencies most want to see treated, and to indicate this to those concerned. At the same time he must realise and sympathise with the concern and bewilderment and apprehension which the child's behaviour occasions.

### 5. Working with the social services

This is a very important role, which may at times involve the whole clinic team. It is expected that the child psychiatrist will have sessions in community homes and assist at assessment centres, and that he will have many fruitful meetings with his colleagues in the social service department to discuss matters of mutual interest (as well as families) and to formulate plans for joint enterprises.*

The work of the social service department is inevitably different from the work of the clinic. The department must accept allcomers the clinic may choose, the department, because of statutory duties, is forced at times to 'intrude' on families and act coercively, the clinic may protect families under the cloak of confidentiality, and so on.

Yet there is no excuse for the 'them' and 'us', 'thine' and 'mine' attitude. Problems overlap as well as diverge, and it is feasible as well as desirable for the two settings to work together, with a family, where there is neglect or damage to a child or children, the clinic psychotherapist or social worker may work with the mother and child together, drawing them closer through shared play, while the social worker from the department may work with the father, siblings or with the whole family. Or again the social worker from the department may join the child psychiatrist in family interviews held at the clinic or at the department.

It is also most beneficial for clinics and social service departments to mount joint enterprises, such as shared adolescent groups for teenagers, meetings with groups of teachers, or combined study days.

*The setting up of 'nurture groups' is described on p. 41, footnote.

The psychiatrist's contribution in assessment centres is important, and in community homes essential as well as rewarding. Mutual support may enable the two working groups to do what neither could do alone (Donnison([12])), to keep a family together, to prevent frequent and perhaps unnecessary admissions of young children to hospital or to convalescent homes or to check the progress of an adolescent down the slippery slope to delinquency by a combined approach to the problem.

### 6. Prevention*

It could be claimed that the whole child guidance movement is geared to prevention, especially with the present-day emphasis on the treatment of young children, and of families, and the work done by the Robertsons and others (with its attendant publicity) on the humanisation of paediatric wards, and on separation. As a greater understanding of disadvantage and deprivation develops, here again children and their parents may receive an understanding kind of help which will prevent further damage to relationships and persons.

Prevention and primary care are big news today. Starting prior to birth, 'at risk' mothers may be picked out at antenatal clinics or in their families or at a later stage immediately after the birth. Support and on-going casework may be offered to these mothers either through the health visitor or midwife or through clinic social workers who are working with them. Attention is being focused on 'high risk areas' at infant welfare clinics, where feeding, sleeping and other handling problems are rife in families where young children have been born in rapid succession, and/or to young and immature parents; or where both parents are working to struggle to attain or maintain the standards of their neighbours. Here it is common for unfavourable relationships to develop between mothers (and fathers) and the young children and for the situation to become deadlocked.

Help may be offered in a number of ways; one is a toddlers' group run by the health visitor, with a mother's group organised concurrently by another health visitor or a clinic social worker. Or mothers may be invited to bring their pre-school children to the child guidance clinic, where parallel groups are offered with the toddler going to the psychotherapist, and the mother to the social worker. Long-term, on-going caring casework is usually required for the mothers, especially for those who have been deprived themselves, with the aim not only of improving interaction with the child who is showing

*See Caplan.([14,15])

problems, but to strengthen the chances of better relationships with subsequent children.

The work done on paediatric wards with the mothers of young babies admitted with problems of management or development, or in cases on non-accidental injury to the child, fall into the same category. For these young children and for slightly older children, special centres have been set up in a number of areas, where the needs of these children and their families are provided for by a team of workers, usually on a day basis. Such a centre has been functioning for the past four years at the Hospital for Sick Children, Great Ormond Street, London (Bentovim[13])).

Child guidance developed piecemeal and in all sorts of holes and corners, under all sorts of authorities and with varied orientations. For these and other reasons it tended originally to be rather isolated and mysterious. It is a welcome change that we are being encouraged to look outwards even more than we have been striving to do of late, both to medical colleagues and to the community, particularly to the social service departments, and to educational establishments of all kinds.

If child psychiatrists are to be accepted as well as useful, and they can scarcely be useful if they are not accepted, we must make certain that avenues of communication are kept open and free from bias and prejudice, and from polarisation into 'We' and 'You'. Time and again the patient, whether child or family, suffers because of failures of communication and lack of mutual understanding between those who want to help the child. There are many examples of this in this book. A clear understanding of what the child psychiatrist can and cannot do is the first requisite and in my view he should be willing, to get out of the clinic in order to demonstrate this, if necessary with part or all of his clinic team.

## Bibliography and Further Reading

Items marked * are particularly important sources. Unnumbered references provide alternative sources to the reference quoted immediately above.

1.  Anthony, S. (1940) *The Child's Discovery of Death,* Kegan Paul, Trench, Trubner Co., London.
2.  Woodward, J. and Jackson, D. (1961) Emotional reactions in burned children and their mothers, *Br. J. plast. Surg.* **13,** 316–324.
3.  Caplan, G. (ed.) (1961) *Prevention of Mental Disorders in Children,* Tavistock Publications, London.

4. Irvine, E. (1959) The use of small group discussions in the teaching of human relations and mental health, *Br. J. Psychiat. Soc. Work* **5**, 1, 26–30.

5. Balint, M. (1957) *The Doctor, his Patient and the Illness*, Pitman Medical Publications, London.

6. Levitt, E. (1955) The effect of a causal teacher training program on authoritarianism and responsibility in grade school children, *Psychol. Rep.* **1**, 449–458.

7. Isaac, N. H. (1958) The formation of a teachers' group, *Br. J. Psychiat. Soc. Work* **4**, 3, 18–22.

8. Smith, J. (1957) An experiment in consultation, *Br. J. Psychiat. Soc. Work* **4**, 2, 16–20.

9. Meyer, V. and Chesser, E. S. (1970) *Behaviour Therapy in Clinical Psychiatry*, Penguin Books, Harmondsworth.

10. Moore, E. M. (1961) School visits: the role of phantasy, *J. Child Psychol. Psychiat.* **2**, 2, 127–135.

11. Skynner, A. C. R. (1971) The 'minimum sufficient network', *Social Work Today* **3**, 9, 3–7.

12. Donnison, D. (1954) *The Neglected Child and the Social Services*, Manchester University Press, Manchester.

13. Bentovim, A. (1973) *Disturbed and under-5 Special Education*, Spastics Society, London.

*14. Caplan, G. (1961) *An Approach to Community Mental Health*, Tavistock Publications, London.

15. Caplan, G. (1964) *Principles of Preventive Psychiatry*, Tavistock Publications, London.
    Gath, D. (1968) Child Guidance and the general practitioner, *J. Child Psychol. Psychiat.* **9**, 3/4, 213–227.

# Name Index

# Subject Index